THE SPIRITUAL JOURNEY WITH BELL'S PALSY

How to Overcome Your Condition to Have an Abundance of Health

Bernice Gayle

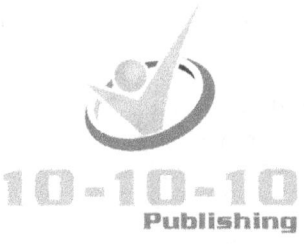

The Spiritual Journey with Bell's Palsy:
How to overcome your condition to have an abundance of health
Gayle, Bernice

Copyright © 2018 by Bernice Gayle

ISBN-13: 978-1727239041
ISBN-10: 1727239040

No part of this publication may be reproduced, stored in a retrieval system or transmitted in any form or by any means, electronic, mechanical, photocopying, recording, scanning or otherwise.

All rights reserved, including the right to reproduce this book or portions thereof in any form whatsoever.

Published by:
10-10-10 Publishing
Markham, Ontario

First 10-10-10 Publishing paperback edition July 2018

Contents

Dedication	v
Foreword	vii
Acknowledgements	ix
Chapter 1: The Disturbance	**1**
A Quick Thing	1
The Mask Of Deceptions	3
Searching	4
Not Knowing, The Unknown	5
Assessments	6
Exchange Of Energy	9
Chapter 2: The Journey	**11**
Weakness In The Body	11
What Is Bell's Palsy?	13
Who Is Charles Bell?	14
Earache	15
When My Smile Decided To Park	16
Inflammations In The Body	17
Chapter 3: Spiritualism	**19**
Life Balance	19
The Body With A View	22
Be Authentic	23
Spiritual Awakening	26
Accept Yourself	28
Trust Yourself	33

Chapter 4: Meditation — 37
What Is Meditation? — 37
Mind, Body, And Soul — 40
What Is The Spirit? — 43
How To Stay Focused? — 44
Opening Your Third Eye — 47
Healing Through Visualisation — 51
Grounded — 53

Chapter 5: Beyond Who You Are — 55
Stop Holding Onto The Past — 55
What Is Your True Self? — 57
Affirmation — 59
A Moment For Reflection — 62
How To Accept Change — 64
Being In Harmony With Nature — 66
Depleted Soils — 67

Chapter 6: The Awakening — 69
Self-Fulfilment — 69
Happiness — 70
Joy — 71
Ideas And Realities — 72
Accepting An Emotion — 72

Chapter 7: The Unquiet Mind — 75
Worrying About Worrying — 75
Keeping Worries To Yourself — 76
Emotional Reactions — 77
Your Values — 78
Powerful Autopilot — 79
Uncertainty

Chapter 8: Transformation   81
What Is Transformation?   81
Gratitude   **82**
Reality Versus Illusion   82
Diving Deep   83
Be Selfish   84
Negative Visualisation   **84**
Encouragement From Mother Earth   85

Chapter 9: Recovery   87
Temporary Weakness   87
The Onset   88
Within 9 Months   89
Exercise   90

Chapter 10: Your Health Is Your Wealth   93
Holistic Health   93
What Is Health?   94
Wealth   95
Healing The Body Through Music   95
Healthy Food   97
Food To Avoid   98

About The Author   101

I dedicate this book to my grandmother, Grandma Aunty Jenny, who had shaped my thinking, and was always with me during my spiritual journey whilst writing this book. You are my inspiration.

Foreword

Are you in control of your life? Do you realise that you have the POWER within you to SUCCEED?

In *The Spiritual Journey With Bell's Palsy,* author Bernice Gayle's intention is to help you understand that you can achieve more success.

Having an illness or a serious disease can drastically change your situation or circumstance, and can have an impact of who you were and who you have become. No matter where you are at this juncture in your life, you can change your decisions, and change your future.

Through the pages of this book, Bernice will encourage you to challenge your ways of life, find your moral values, guide your life accordingly, and learn to be your authentic self.

You must be truthful with yourself to overcome challenges or obstacles that are preventing you from being your unique self without compromise. By being truthful to yourself and others, you will find huge power and success.

Raymond Aaron
New York Times Bestselling Author

Acknowledgements

I would like to thank my son, **Leon Gayle**, for being my rock when I was doing very poorly. It was his strength and encouragement that kept me going, and helped me stay focused, regardless of the changes that my whole body was going through. Looking at my face every morning, and asking me to carry out certain actions, like raising my eyebrows, are things that I will always hold onto for the rest of my life. To have a son like **Leon Gayle**, I am truly blessed in every way.

I am grateful for having **Andrea Gayle**, my daughter, who was always in the background and making sure that I was comfortable, even when I was far from being in that state. I deeply appreciate the endless moments when she would sit with me, and we would share our events of the day together. It's very uplifting, especially when at times I was so weak to discuss ideas. She knew I was not my usual self but kept quiet, and when I was ready to talk, she too was ready. I give thanks to my son, **Colin Barnett,** for our long and deep conversations on the phone.

Thanks to my brothers, especially **Lambert McCook and Afton Mc Cook**. They were always at the end of the phone, almost every day, to check on how I was progressing. At times, **Lambert McCook** would leave whatever he was doing to be by my side and make sure that I was having my *belly full* of laughter as part of my medications to aid my recovery. Both my brothers showed me the endless love that we had always had for each other, and it will never, never stop.

I would like to thank my mum, **Rose McCook**, for choosing me out of all the other thousands of eggs. My achievements and successes would not have been fulfilled without her.

My acknowledgement goes to my sister, **Judith Barnett**, whose messages were always refreshing and loving, and my cousin, **Claudette Walker**, and her husband, **Frank**. Despite the time of the day, they were constantly on the phone from Jamaica to hear my voice. **Judith Barnett** said, on several occasions, "If I don't hear from you, my soul is not at peace." Having such remarkable members of my family showed me how grateful I am to have them in my life.

The other people who were significant during my spiritual journey were my grandchildren; especially, **Shai Gayle**, **Meshach Gayle-Swell**, and **Isaiah Gayle-Swell**. They were great at talking and listening to me when I explained my feelings. They were true warriors.

I would like to thank **Michael Gayle** for being himself.

I am honoured to have **Dr. A. Adeyeye,** at the Honor Oak Group Practice, who treated and supported me throughout my condition with Bell's palsy. It was **Dr. A. Adeyeye's** energy, together with her expertise, that put my mind at ease, especially when I was *down in the dumps*.

Acknowledgements

Thanks to my publisher, **Raymond Aaron**, for his commitment and support and encouragement to trust my own style of writing. He taught me so much about the fundamental principles of being an author, and the benefit of being an authority in branding. I was very happy to know that someone like him was nearby to walk me through the steps.

I would like to extend a huge thank you to my local radio station, Galaxyafiwe, especially one of the main presenters, **Aboo Rahtata**, who has a loving and warm heart to work *in the box*, *out of the box*, and to go that extra mile for his community.

I would like to extend my gratitude to **Adrian Uden**, from whom I learnt that opportunities for change come in all shapes and sizes in life, and that sometimes they may even seem more like tragedies than opportunities. An acute or a chronic illness, or loss of a dream, can act as a catalyst to help us break out of that tiny box we all create to stay in. It was not until the challenges of life's journey that **Adrian Uden** showed me, and from which I realise, life is truly a gift. Being who he is, I was able to listen carefully to messages within and without, to further help guide me to my authentic self.

Lastly, but most importantly, my greatest gratitude goes to my **Higher Power**, the **Creator,** for taking me along this spiritual journey and giving me the courage, strength, and determination to accomplish this walk.

Chapter 1

The Disturbance

"My attitude has always been, if you fall flat on your face, at least you're moving forward. All you have to do is get back up and try again."
Richard Branson

A Quick Thing

You are reading this because you, a family member, or a friend has been diagnosed with Bell's palsy. This is often called facial palsy, or facial paralysis.

Does your life seem to be out of control at this moment? Are there times when you feel as if you cannot go on anymore? Where can you go for help? Do you feel as if you are being run by your life? I know you are thinking deeply about the questions I posed. Let me tell you how I felt in this modern and complex world we live in. Come and walk with me!

I was feeling very, very unwell for months, maybe for a period of almost 2 years. Every so often, I was feeling weak, and I was not sure what the problem was. At times, I felt as if I was going to pass out, either early in the morning or during the day. WOW! WOW! On several occasions, coming down the stairs, at work or at home, made me very weak, as if I was on my way to passing out.

I was still feeling sick within my whole body. The feeling of weakness was getting worse, but I carried on working as a primary school teacher. Feeling this way was not helping my situation, because as soon as I reached home, especially when I arrived late, I was greeted with bad looks from Guy, whom I lived with. I carried on teaching as a supply teacher, which was my way out of my situations.

After being in Luton for two years, I felt I had made the biggest mistake ever. But that was a chance I took. Had I taken the time to find out more about Guy, then maybe I would not have felt the way I did, or the way I still do. Moving to Luton was a quick thing. Again, I did not carry out a thorough search on the area but just went with Guy on his trips to visit his brother. Seeing a part of it whilst the visits, I liked what I had seen. I had spoken to two people about the place, and they gave me some good reviews, such as a good place to live. That helped me to make my mind up. But then I didn't explore their ideas of the meaning of *good*. Going to Luton was also a way of me getting out of London. I must say, my head teacher in London at the time did not like Luton when I told her I wanted to move there. She did not give any reason to justify it. I just thought she didn't want me to leave her school because I was one of her senior managers.

The Mask Of Deceptions

Over a period, I thought the man, whom I had moved into my house, started to slowly *shed the mask from his face*, with his verbal abuses and his emotional looks, and was hiding the fact that he was an alcoholic. He was drinking and smoking heavily. It was hard for me to see him like that. Even with the abuse from him, I begged him to stop. He said he couldn't just stop like that. It was tearing me apart. I must say I was biding my time. It was only a matter of time; I was waiting for the opportunity to do something.

I was still feeling unwell all over my body, and not knowing what to do or whom to turn to for help. Because I was feeling so unwell, I phoned the herbalist, but he was not answering my calls. I texted him on numerous occasions, but he had not responded. Getting no reply from him, I stopped taking his supplements and decided to carry out some research on the internet. I looked at all the symptoms that I was having, but most of them were saying the same things. I spoke to someone in one of the biggest health shops, and she suggested vitamins and other natural remedies, but I was still feeling unwell.

Being so exhausted, I went to one of the walk-in clinics in Luton, about three times. On my final visit, I told the doctor that during the night I felt so bad I thought I was going to die. When he asked me why I felt that way, I outlined in depth how I felt during the night: being very weak. He suggested for me to see my GP. When I visited my GP, I told her about my feelings, and that I had changed my eating habits by not adding things like salt when I cooked. More blood and urine tests were carried out, together with having a nerve ultrasound. The results of that was normal, but I was feeling worse, to the point that I wanted to pass out.

Searching

During the summer holidays, I thought seriously about whether I should work for four days, but decided I did not want to do that, because my health was still not to my satisfaction. I made the choice to stay off work for a while. I kept my promise and worked on ME. Despite not working in schools, I was still going to Luton and London to tutor a group of children.

Whilst in London, I received a text message from Guy, asking me to let him know where in London I was living because the council noted that my address was in Luton. I did not understand the text message because both of us knew that I was living in Luton but staying in London. I told him that I would talk with him but only when he was sober. These words were often repeated by me to him. When I asked him about the letter, he said the council had evidence that I lived in Luton.

It was then that I told him on the phone that I was not sure what he was talking about because, as far as I was concerned, I was living in Luton. It was then that he said I had been living in London for the past three years. That got me because, up until September of 2017, I had worked and lived in Luton. It was a shock to hear something like that coming from Guy's mouth. When I told him that the addresses of all the schools I had been working at were documented and that I had started to work in London in October 2017, I noticed, at my house, things for someone who needed walking aids were beginning to appear in the house, together with a high chair in the kitchen. Walking sticks were stacked away in the corner of one of the rooms, and there was a support for getting in and out of the bath. I was not sure where this was going, and it did not look good. I was very SAD.

Not Knowing, The Unknown

I had a bad earache, which was painful. Despite this, I was able to eat some lovely fish with vegetables that my daughter, Andrea, had cooked on Tuesday night. During the night, I felt that my mouth didn't feel right. Knowing her and how she loved experimenting with her food, it was then that I thought she might have put some different spices in the fish, which was causing a reaction. When I spoke to Leon, my son, he said that his mouth also felt a bit weird, so he put some cream on it. According to him, it worked.

Later, I went off to sleep for a short while. When I woke up, Leon said that I had been sleeping with my left eye wide open. I smiled and made a joke out of it. It was then that I asked Andrea if she had put any other spices in the fish. When I told her that my mouth felt unusually funny, she said she had only put the same natural seasoning in the fish.

In the morning, when I was brushing my teeth, my face did not look right. It was leaning to the right, and I couldn't wash my mouth out without the water going everywhere. It was then that I began to get very worried and nervous, so I went straight to the GP, before 7am. I was seen by the doctor at about 8:15am. Whilst in the room, I told her that I felt as if I was having a stroke. She looked at me and said, "You look very pale." It was then that she took my blood pressure and said it was very high: 187/100. Soon, she investigated my ears and said the left one was inflamed, and she suggested that I go straight to Lewisham hospital to have an ECG, blood tests, and a urine test. She gave me the address of an optician for an eye test. I did all of these on the same day.

The doctor prescribed some antibiotics and ear drops. After my visit to the hospital, and collecting my medications, I went home and fell off to sleep after taking them. Andrea came from work, at about 4pm, and was on the phone. When she asked if I was okay, I told her that I felt as though I was having a stroke, and was about to phone for an ambulance. Immediately, she hung up the phone and was speaking to me as I sat on the settee. She looked at me and was quite worried to see me in the state that I was in. It was then that she phoned the emergency services. She got through and asked for the ambulance. At that moment, I knew she was very worried. It showed on her face. Although I was worried and anxious, I felt as though what was happening to me right now was in the making. Finally, my health problems that had been causing all the bad feelings in me were coming out. My, oh my!

Assessments

When they were talking to Andrea on the phone, she was asked to carry out several exercises on me. Whatever they asked her to do, she echoed for me to carry them through. Once they were satisfied, they hung up, and Andrea asked me to remain on the settee without moving, but I moved to get something that I needed from my hang bag. Eventually, the ambulance crew arrived. They were very quick. There was one woman and two men. They carried out the same exercises that Andrea did with me. I was asked to raise my eyebrows. It felt as if I was raising both. The other task they asked me to carry out was to raise my hands above my head. One of the crew asked me to try to push down his hands away from him. Then I was asked to poke my tongue out, close my eyes tightly, and to puff my cheeks out, together with showing my teeth. These were difficult for me to do. We take things for granted, until they are no longer functional, and then we realise how fragile our body is.

My blood pressure was constantly being monitored because it was extremely high. It was 180/100. Once they had finished their routine tasks, we went out of the living room, straight to the ambulance. I walked to where they had parked, which was not too far from where I was staying. Two vehicles were there: a paramedic car and an ambulance. Before they started their written assessments, the woman asked me what happened. I then told them the chain of events that took place after I ate my dinner and brushed my teeth, right up to the time I woke up and went to the doctor. I mentioned the fact that the doctor was mostly concerned about how pale I looked, and how high my blood pressure was. They were shocked that the doctor did not carry out any of the exercises they did on me. Andrea and I looked at each other as if to say, "How could the doctor not observe me more closely than she did?"

Sitting on the metal chair whilst being in the hospital was extremely uncomfortable. I was feeling very sick and weak. Later, the doctor called my name and asked me to follow him into a room. Andrea came with me. He asked me to explain how I was feeling. I did. It was then that he carried out the same exercises as the crew from the ambulance. He diagnosed me as having Bell's palsy, and it was going to leave some disabilities. I looked at him and refused to accept his narrative on the disabilities he was talking about.

In my mind, I was saying to myself that I would find people who had or were having such an injury as mine. I would also research as much as I could about it. It was then that I turned to the doctor and said, "That's your opinion, and I refuse to make it real by allowing it to be a self-fulfilling prophecy." Susan Jeffers pointed this out by saying "...the possibility of the unexpected sets us up for a great deal of fear. We anticipate the worst." Yes, I accepted what had happened to me but refused to allow it to *disable* my mind. Although my body was weak, and my face felt as if it was swelling, I had my inner strength to talk.

All I wanted was to go home and sleep. The doctor told us he had prescribed some medications. One, he said, was steroids. It was an anti-inflammatory called Prednisolone, with a dosage of 5mg, to reduce both swelling and inflammation. He suggested for me to take it in the mornings for seven days. The other one was also to reduce the swelling, on the left side of my face. It was an antiviral medicine to prevent the virus from multiplying. It was almost 9pm, and he told us to be quick because the pharmacy was about to close. We got there on time. In no time, we arrived at home. I took one of the tablets and went off to sleep.

Exchange Of Energy

Shortly, I was fully awake but lying down. Being unable to sleep, my heart was beating rapidly, and lots of things in my body felt as if they were at war with each other. I had never had or felt this experience in my whole body. I was getting worried and anxious, but I tried to keep still and work with what was going on in my body. During the activities going on in my body, I was sweating and was in extreme pain. The pain was mostly in my left ear. To get comfortable, I was twisting and turning in the hope of getting relief from the pain. It was not happening. When I looked in the mirror, my mouth was twisted to the right, and my lips were swollen, as well as my left cheek. I did not recognise ME. At this point, I wanted to cry but couldn't. It's like my tears had dried out.

It was now early morning and my family was awake. I tried to brush my teeth but could not because the pain was unbearable. I used my finger to gentle move my lips to try cleaning my teeth. Although it was difficult, I managed. Washing out my mouth with water was very problematic. I had to clench my fist and gently put it to my mouth, then swish it out. To drink from a cup or a glass, I had to use a straw. Eating was very difficult because chewing was painful, so I had to take my time. It took me three times as long now to finish off my meal than before. The medications were making me drowsy, so I was mostly relaxing but couldn't sleep.

It was night time, and I was beginning to feel sleepy. In my sleep, I had a dream where I was in a beautiful green garden with a close friend. We were together, holding hands and constantly talking and playing, like we were young children again. Feeling the way that I had was magnificent. In my dream, I was exhausted, and he knew that, so he slowly put me on the floor of green grass to lie down, and he started to fan me with a large pine leaf. It was so vivid, as if it was real. Having such a dream, Kevin Dorival tells me that *"the essence of healing rituals is based on the belief that an exchange of energy occurs to facilitate healing between two people near each other and the belief that healing will occur."* Part 2 will take you further on my journey. Come along with me to discover things that I saw whilst travelling.

Chapter 2

The Journey

"You may not always have a comfortable life, and you will not always be able to solve all of the world's problems at once, but don't ever underestimate the importance you can have, because history has shown us that courage can be contagious, and hope can take on a life of its own."
Michelle Obama

Weakness In The Body

Is this a part of my courage? Come along so that I can take you with me to my place of hope. I am going to remind you of the condition that, for me, was mysterious. Are there mechanisms? What are they?

It's important at this juncture to look at some of the biological mechanisms that lead to my disease, known as Bell's palsy. The condition is rare. Let us look closely at the labelled diagram below. From this, we can see that the myelin sheath is protecting the nerve fibres in the brain, the optic nerves, and the spinal cord. This is a thin covering like the layer of an onion. This myelin sheath does not cover the whole nerve but in segments, leaving tiny gaps, called Nodes of Ranvier. The tiny gaps are like a two-terminal electrical component that stores potential energy in an electric field. It charges and allows bursts of electric impulses to move along the neuron easily. Our cells have cytoplasm. It is a clear fluid that fills the inside of the cell and surrounds all the internal structures.

Because its fluid is a gel-like appearance, it contains strands of proteins for holding the cell's internal parts in place. Doing this, it looks after nutrition, like salt and chemicals such as enzymes for the cell. The cytoplasm is necessary to support the cell. It provides movement like hormones and gets rid of waste products from the cell; however, it does not move things. We can look at the cell nucleus as its brain. It regulates the functions of the cell to process information. Dendrites are like trees with branches. They receive electrical messages from the axons of neurons so that the cells can become active. I want you to imagine that you widen this gap.

This slows the nerve impulse, or might even stop it, which leads to neurological problems because you get a blocked conduction block. Now, you cannot get the full use of that nerve, leaving you with weakness in the body. I forgot to tell you about the axon. I want you to think of it as if the whole neuron is cut. The result of this is that the axonal degeneration occurs, which will then produces severe paralysis. Since this conduction block happens nearer its origin, we usually see a rapid and complete recovery in about 85%, from onset of the condition. Knowing this, let us turn to examine Bell's palsy.

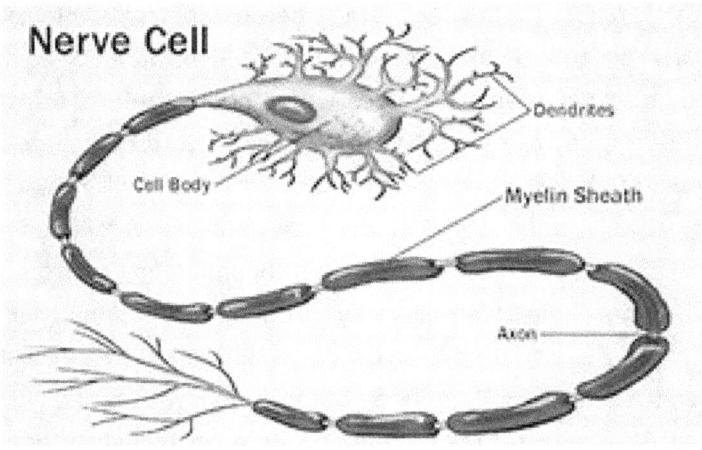

What Is Bell's Palsy?

Bell's palsy is a condition that causes temporary weakness of the muscles in the face. The cause of it is not fully known. Some researchers say that it is likely caused by a virus, usually herpes, which seems to inflame the nerves. In addition to this, the herpes virus is the one that also causes cold sores and genital herpes. It is also said that the chickenpox and shingles viruses are linked to Bell's palsy. The question to ask is, what is herpes?

There are several types of herpes viruses. An example is the neonatal herpes simplex virus. This type is rare but can be serious. This is where a mother of a new born baby can transmit the herpes virus to her child. This can be transmitted through kissing a baby whist having a cold sore. The commonly known virus is *herpes*, and this can be highly contagious. It is spread by skin-to-skin contact during sexual intercourse, or even by just a kiss.

Let me go back to the idea that the herpes virus is likely to cause Bell's palsy. Because children from the age of ten might not be actively engaged in sexual intercourse, they would not, therefore, transmit herpes. During my research, Llaila O. Afrika showed that there is a biochemical imbalance in such things as birth control pills, bleach in sanitary towels, and so on. In this case, the body rejected the chemicals, which can take months to rid the inflammation from the body. Therefore, the body will always produce herpes whenever it's trying to cleanse itself from toxins. "When this happens," as Llaila O. Afrika continued to say, "The body becomes mildly or severely sick, and eventually collapses the immunity system, resulting in diseases." I was doing very poorly for a few days.

Who Is Charles Bell?

The name, Bell's palsy, is said to be named after a Scottish man, Charles Bell, from the 19th Century. He was a surgeon and a neurologist who studied the structure of various branches of the body. With this in mind, Charles Bell established that the nerves of the special senses could be traced from certain areas of the brain to the organs. Because of his knowledge and skills, he is noted for discovering the difference between sensory nerves and motor nerves in the spinal cord. He is noted to be the first person for describing the condition of Bell's palsy. In view of this, Charles Bell believed that a cranial nerve, in the face, controlled muscles of expression. The symptom can start one or two weeks after a cold, an eye infection, or in my case, an ear infection that came on very suddenly.

Earache

Any damage to the facial nerves travels through a narrow, bony canal in the skull, beneath the ear, to the muscles on each side of the face. Because of this, most of the nerve's journey is encased in the bony shell of the skull. The sensory hair cells of the ear nerve can get damaged by ear infections. Injury to the bone can cause damage to the nerve in the ear, resulting in earache.

I can't remember ever having an earache, but suddenly, it happened to me. I had heard of people with earaches, and the most common thing they said was that you should avoid smoking, which I had never signed up for. The other thing they would say was to avoid exposure to second hand smokers. How can you do this? Finally, they would say that allergy triggers, like dust and pollen, can irritate your sinuses, which can cause earaches.

Having this earache felt like when you are taking a spoonful of honey from a jar. It was heavy and sticky. Wherever I turned, it was getting more and more heavy and sticky. The pain was unbearable and uncontrollable. It felt as if it was coming from the back of my ear, towards my brain, every few seconds. Then I would feel a shooting volt of pain that went to the back of my head. Then, my left ear started to ring. I thought it might have been part of the motor and sensory components that enters the bone close to my inner ear. Although it was worrying, it was for a short period of time.

At times, the pain felt like I needed to get a stick to scratch it. The feeling was terrible. What I did was to focus on staying still for a moment. Doing this allowed me to let go of whatever bad thoughts I had going through my mind, I buried them. Being still also gave myself a space emotionally and physically to make sure that I was using my energy to create a balance. This takes me on to the next part of my journey, where my smile decided to park.

When My Smile Decided To Park

Things were happening to my face. When I was talking, my top lip had a pop-like vibration. I was talking with my mouth moving to the right of my face. I was trying to smile, but it was not happening. The left side of my face was still sore and swollen after a month of suffering from Bell's palsy. Although I was constantly observing my face in the mirror, it was worrying to see the condition. Being a primary school teacher, I was always smiling with my learners whilst teaching. To see my teeth not showing at all, I felt that maybe the doctor was correct when he said it was going to leave me with some disabilities.

The features of my face were stiff. I was unable to open my mouth completely without experiencing lots of discomfort. I was still unable to raise my left eyebrow, together with closing my eye. Trying to smile and show all my teeth was still not possible because my left side refused to move. It was not a great sight, especially if you are a person like me who likes smiling.

In my case, no matter how hard I tried to smile, my brain was sending messages but my face was in a silent mode, and I couldn't smile. It made me realise that having a wide smile is a precious thing to treasure.

Inflammations In The Body

Most of us know that inflammation causes a lot of our health issues, and some of us know how and what to do to further reduce everyday inflammation.

The main physical symptoms that a lot of us suffer from is inflammation. Our body is great at healing itself, but when this is not happening for a period, it's a result of excessive free radical activity and tissue damage. We need to know what free radicals are. When an oxygen molecule splits into single atoms with unpaired electrons, they are called free radicals. If the electrons are not in pairs, free radicals will act as scavengers to seek out other electrons so they can become a pair. The results of this might cause problems, such as damage to cells, proteins, and the nucleic acid instructional code, which may cause the new cells to grow incorrectly.

But then, we have substances in our body, such as antioxidants, that can prevent free radicals from taking electrons and causing damage. Antioxidants are natural substances in the body, and can work with an electron by giving it a free radical without becoming unstable; therefore, stopping a chain reaction from occurring. Just like when our house needs cleaning and we clear the waste, similarly, the antioxidants' job is to clean up the free radical waste in the cells. We are familiar with beta-carotene, vitamin C, and vitamin E: these are antioxidants. Where there is an imbalance, free radicals can damage our cells, which can cause diseases. Having said that, we have substances that can generate free radicals, which can be found in the food we eat, the medicines we take, the air we breathe, and the water we drink.

In addition to the free radicals damaging our cells, surely the body is able to turn air and food into chemical energy. Does that mean they have an important role to play? It depends on a chain reaction of free radicals. Free radicals play a vital part in the immune system because they float through the veins and attack any foreign invaders.

Chapter 3

Spiritualism

"Every man lives in two realms: the internal and the external. The internal is that realm of spiritual ends expressed in art, literature, morals…..The external is that complex of devices, techniques, mechanisms, and instrumentalities by means of which we live."
Martin Luther King Jr

Life Balance

I know my body is a direct reflection of everything I do in my life. It is the physical manifestation of my inner self in terms of who am I. Having said that, healing of my body, mind, and soul comes with my understanding of how I balanced everything in my life.

Reading various reports, together with my experiences I outlined in previous parts, there is an understanding that Bell's palsy is of an emotional component. The reactivation of the viruses that I discussed, such as herpes and shingles, may be the underlying cause of Bell's palsy. Some of us know that when the body is going through periods of stress, viruses can erupt.

Does that mean that I was going through a period of stress at a very young age, to adulthood? Let me tell you a story from my childhood, of putting my emotional component to the test.

At a young age, maybe at the age of 5, I remember being with my Grandma Aunty Jenny, whilst in Jamaica. Everyone called her Aunty Jenny, regardless of their social status. I was always with her. I loved her dearly. Sticking to her like glue gave me some strong lessons, which I treasured. She was a vendor who worked in one of the top markets, called Coronation Market. It was busy and colourful, and the noise was buzzing, because vendors were calling customers to buy their goods. Coronation Market was the largest farmer's market, where vendors from all over the island would go to sell their fresh produce. I often wondered why it was called Coronation Market. In 1739, it was the heart of Jamaica's commerce.

She would give me goods to sell in and out of the market. At a tender age, she would say to me, "Make sure everything is sold before you get back. You are going to work hard for your living." Yes, I was nervous then. Now, looking back, I know she was preparing me for my life's journey, and it was meant to be second to none. I had to look at what was working for her. I asked myself questions back then: How did she get customers to buy her goods? What was her attitude towards them? I had to process all these things to build on, so that the things that she gave me to sell would have been sold before my journey back to her. Being prepared like this, at a tender age, enabled me to think quickly to accomplish my given tasks.

Spiritualism

No matter what had been thrown at me, I had to prepare myself. Doing this would take me to the next level for my vision in life. Because Grandma Aunty Jenny prepared me from an early age, I knew I would be unstoppable. My mind-set, in terms of my emotions, was to feel guilty if I let someone down or they made a promise but never kept it. I must say, I denied some emotions, and they became chronic. An example of this was having deep, deep feelings for a man, who seemed to be on the same *plane* as me, but when I needed his help, he avoided me. Yes, I was very angry, and not sure where to go or whom to speak to. Because I cared a lot about him, the emotional pain was very hard to let go. Being avoided like this, I forgave him. This has taught me a spiritual lesson. My lesson here is to develop my *inner* voice to communicate and to appreciate the impact of his behaviour. I respect his energy, together with others around me.

Did you know you have 43 different muscles in your face, and that a slight change in any of the facial muscles can influence what you are feeling or thinking? Having read my story, does that show I was in denial of my condition with Bell's palsy? From reading a section in the metaphysical literature, they noted that the *"root cause of Bell's palsy is about denying emotions. It is the manifestation of the extreme control over anger, and the unwillingness or inability to express that anger."* Therefore, being unable to recognise an emotion is a result of denial. From this, the anger will then appear on the face and show up as facial paralysis. Surely, you can be angry if you want. If you want to laugh, then you have the right to laugh.

The Body With A View

I have come to understand that it's our habits that determine who we are and what we do in life. The habits that we learn from an early age determine if we are living to our full potential. Let us look at the psychology of life. Today, we are in a world of technology, which gives us lots of information about our health. Some of it might be correct, and some might not be. In this case, we can make a comparison and *filter* the ones that can be harmful to our health.

A lot of us are not truly happy with our health. This is because most people are unconscious: they live on a superficial level of life, which is based on what they observe. The results that they see, they don't like them. How many times have you been to fast-food restaurants and have seen very obese people there, saying, " I am too fat; I need to lose weight?" When you look at them, they are stuffing themselves with greasy food that is full of unsaturated fat and lots of salt, and they are drinking sugary drinks. Many of us will continue to eat this way, and will focus our energy on what is considered as unhealthy food, because it looks good and, at times, tastes good. What is causing the problem? Is it to do with how many people are influenced and shaped from their childhood? This will affect how they think about the *wrong* types of foods, which leads to self-defeating thoughts and habits. "What is invisible is what creates what is visible."

Since we are looking at the things we see and are taught, we respond to the superficial level of life. Therefore, the last place we look to find the results, is within ourselves. I realised that most people's thoughts are holding them back from having good health.

Spiritualism

Looking through the body of *self* can open our eyes to our self-destruction, our habits, and our attitudes. It opens the door to identify the things in our lives that give us a sense of inner peace, comfort, strength, and connection. Looking at the body with this view, revels the strengths that we seek to guide us through health challenges, or any other ones that come our way.

What is the lesson? It's simple. When we know who we are, and understand our habits, each day we learn more about ourselves, and therefore we can support and encourage ourselves to live a healthier life style. It's the way to finding meaning, hope, and comfort, through art, music, or connecting to nature.

Be Authentic

To be authentic, you must be truthful with yourself. You shouldn't be wearing a mask that can't reveal the person you truly are. If, by any chance, you are wearing that mask, it's crucial for you to show your real face, despite the cost.

Saying that does not mean that you need to unmask others. To them, they are happy with telling lies; therefore, it's for them to know that—not you. Here is a story about a person I lived with for 13 years, who was wearing a mask. I decided that I would not unmask this person, because that is how he thinks. I moved out of my house. Occasionally, I would go there to collect my mail and other personal belongings that I might need. Upon arrival, on one of these occasions, when I entered the living room, the air engulfed me with a stale smell of cigarettes.

Eventually, he entered the living room from the kitchen, and looked at me. Searching my face conjured up something, so he started talking about my childhood, which, according to him, I never had. My grandmother raised me from an early age, and to him, it was not up to her to do that. Listening to him going on and on felt like an auto-play. The thing that my inner voice tells me is to hold onto my dreams, and never, never give those up. My grandmother planted this in my mind by saying, "Most people go so far in their lives; then they park themselves." This is so true, because he was wearing the mask, and therefore not looking at the terrible hurts, and some hits, along his path.

To be authentic, you really need to listen to your inner voice and follow your dreams; otherwise, your whole life will be wasted. You will never have fulfilment if you listen to what a certain person wants you to do. I often wonder if he had been sent to me as a *life giver.* Was it a lesson to be taught to me, that right now, I am too gifted and talented to be in such a situation with a man like him? Perhaps he was showing me the light to my greatness, and to avoid hitting the brakes and being parked.

I need to say that sometimes our inner voice can lead us into danger, so it's important to be truthful. In my situation, being with my grandmother from an early age has taught me to be observant. It's my being. Having said this, you must not allow others to manipulate and control your mind. People will want to change you; they will want to give you their direction, even if you did not ask for it. For me, *I am the container and cannot be contained*, because I am the beholder of my blueprint.

Spiritualism

Many of us are told, when growing up, to hide our feelings; that you should laugh when you are angry. Surely, your smile becomes false; therefore, you are wearing a mask. One thing you do get from smiling in this way is exercising your facial muscles. Because you are not being true to yourself, when you do want to smile, you cannot. In this state, your mind is getting conflicting messages, because when you are meant to be angry, you avoid it; therefore, having mixed information does not work. From this, be happy if you want to. Have that big belly laugh—laugh and laugh. To be angry is fine. What is wrong with this? You will come to the realisation that your mind is not being overwhelmed with mixed messages. Being in this state, you are not fearful and being judged. Because of what we are told growing up, we tend to hide our authentic selves to fit in with the crowd, without knowing. The result is that we suppress our creativity and the awareness of who we *truly* are. With modern technology, such as social media, it takes the idea away from being who you are. You are not wholeheartedly expressing your *true self*. It brings us back to wearing a mask.

Before I continue to my next section, I want to draw your attention to this idea of being authentic. An article, from *Philosophy Now*, says:

"Becoming authentic is an individual mission, since each person has their own way of being human, and consequently what is authentic will be different for each individual. Furthermore, personal authenticity is highly contextual, and depends on various social, political, religious and cultural characteristics. But the unique nature of each individual is best seen not in who he is, but in who he becomes, and becoming authentic is a continuous process, not an event. It involves not just knowing oneself, but also recognizing others and the mutual influence between individuals. If the quest for personal authenticity is just for self-fulfilment, then it is individualistic and ego-based; but if it is accompanied with the awareness of others and the wider world, then it can be a worthwhile goal."

Spiritual Awakening

When I heard the saying, "Actions speak louder than words," I thought I knew exactly what it meant. No! Before I begin, I must say, it's so very dangerous to put people, or an individual, in a *box,* and give them a label. Spiritual awakening is just the start of a new journey, so that you can see more clearly. This comes through knowledge and understanding of oneself, with the flow of movement we identify as energy. I had a close friend who I knew was not telling the truth. He was dishonest. There was a motive for his behaviour. Why do I say this? His story was always shifting from one thing to the next. Although he was telling me the same story that he had told me less than a week before, it just seemed odd. He was acting out his lies through having sex. He had lots of issues, which he tried to cover up.

Often, he would blame and judge others. When I talked with him, he would say that he was very spiritual. Clearly, the issues regarding himself were not resolved. If we say we are working to help people as an activist, but not knowing the *self,* it will continuously pull us back to the level where the needs are not achieved. They must be met in order to move on. Instead, he was living in a state of fear, anger, and hurt, but appeared to reach peace and joy. Is this, then, his way to grow in a conscious way? I think it is dangerous to work like this

Spiritualism

because his *lower self* is against his *higher self*. He did the correct things, like calling upon his ancestors, doing the right work for the local community, and showing himself as having the right image for people to identify with him.

In my case, speaking with my friend and searching and probing the reality of my spiritual awakening through an ancient African wisdom, I was extremely compulsive. I didn't know what I was looking for or where to go in search of whatever I wanted. Because my friend is an African man, and he grew up on the continent, I was searching his soul for a hint of my quest. It did not happen. He started to tell me about his father being a high priest, and things that my friend had to go through. Because of his stories, which were not convincing, I didn't take in what he was sharing with me as my way into my soul. The inner child within me was quite bruised and needed a lot of healing. My quest was to fill that empty void within my *inner spirit*. Let me make this clear; my searching was not for my friend to heal me. Far from it. It was a feeling or a need that I had never identified because I had been sheltered in a similar way when I depended on my parents to take care of me.

I know that a spiritual awakening is felt throughout my body, in various parts, like my heart, my mind, and my soul. As soon as this phenomenal feeling happened, then I knew I had been taking things less seriously. For me, the feeling was like a *flash of light* that touched deep into my overall being. Because I experienced this, not everyone will go through it in the same way I did. Having a spiritual awakening, the truth within me revealed many things, and my life altered during the process. Having been in this process, I know that my mind is sharper than how it was in the past. I can see things in a realistic way, and not through a *false lens*. I have a profound sense of calm, and I am peaceful, using my energy that moves me intellectually.

Many things used to worry me a lot, and I often wonder why I was being so sensitive to what might have been very trivial, yet it was serious to me. As I now appreciate the basic things of life, like being truthful to myself and having integrity with others around me, it also enabled me to let go of things that had caused me the feeling of pain, so I now embrace it.

A possible definition of having a spiritual awakening is a sudden shift in consciousness. For me, it's like when you are in the bathroom, naked, and about to go into the water. At that moment, you feel a chill in your entire body. That chill is the basis for the spiritual journey, and it can be an empowering feeling. This chill can make you feel that inner space that had never been revealed to you like that, so it's up to you to appreciate it and open to all that it's unfolding. Being in such a state of mind helps us to learn more about who we are becoming. I know that by having a spiritual awakening, I am more disciplined and more focused.

Accept Yourself

Accepting who you are is an ongoing process. It is quite challenging to carry this through because it is not in line with your culture, like technology, values, or money within a family, or the type of education that tells you how you should be. Therefore, the external world can shape your thinking. This is an important area for me because whatever I do, I will always be ME. Even if I tried to improve myself, I am going to be the same person. We can nurture ourselves and accept it. This is a part of the personality, like talents. I see this as the ego. Although it might seem like a static thing, it is not. We need it because of the job that it does in creating an *emotional* drama in our lives. We all need to celebrate our lives on a regular basis, and not just when we are told.

The moment I have thoughts about myself—*I am not good enough; I am not good at Science; I am very smart; I am better than you; are you stupid or what?*—**hearing these statements build my identity; then I begin** to construct my self-image. It is on this basis that I see myself as being *valuable* and strong. Thoughts like these contribute to the structure of the *ego*. While growing up, my ego hid behind the "I" and "me," and to a certain extent, even today. Having the above thoughts, and agreeing with all of them, they define who I am; hence, the reinforcement of the *ego*. For me, problems come into force when I am working on developing ME, especially when the thoughts are not empowering or overly positive. Because I developed lots of values over the years and was not really paying attention, to analyse and turn whatever they were, inward, and notice them, is challenging for me now. Could it be that I am hiding behind my opinions that appear true, and that is what is causing the challenge?

I have had a trail of emotional reactions, either through dreams or thoughts, which resulted in me being angry at my beloved and, at times, wanting to be always right. To accept myself is to accept everything. For this to be strong, I will have to change my beliefs in terms of how I see myself. If, when growing up, you hear that *you are not good enough,* it may conjure up images as to how you should look in order to be accepted. Quite often, my values will offset both my emotions and my personality, so I get very annoyed with myself. Having such feelings and being hard on myself creates the feelings of worthlessness.

To live with this feeling is very painful emotionally, because it hadn't been nurtured. Of course, the pain is masked and covered up. With others watching you, there is the projection that you are happy and full of confidence. But this is not entirely true because you are struggling with the feelings of insecurity and inadequacy, and you are in a state of worthlessness. To raise your inner thoughts and accept who you are, you need to do this in a logical way.

I would like to share the ideas of my inner thoughts through a dream I had. In my dream, the man that I bought my house with rented it without consulting me. Seeing this in my dream was a struggle and very confusing. Being out of my dream, and looking at my inner thoughts, this might have been where I was for many years. It was a way of shutting down by blocking away the pain, although I had my beautiful children around to care for and to love. I had lots of pain, which I could not get rid of. It was like I was looking for something or someone to blame—looking outwards at my dad, whom I did not know, and my mum, when she left my brothers and I in Jamaica for the best parts of our early years.

Being with my mum, at the age of twelve, and living in London, with different cultures, was challenging. The other thing was being in a house where I felt I was the odd one. It felt odd because I was the

Spiritualism

only one with a different surname. Things like this made me valuable and, at the same time, strong, but in serious pain.

I felt like a goldfish in a bowl, searching for belonging. Here, I was the fish in pain, because I was the one amongst many. All I wanted to do was to go back to the environment where I belonged—to be free—instead of being in a small bowl. The thing for me, being in a confined place, was to look deeply at my pain and, therefore, anything that came close to me was insignificant. In a mind-set such as this, I felt I was different due to the fact that I was odd; hence, the pain. Even when I used to walk on the streets and around the corners where boys and men often congregated, my big African backside was something for them to hone in on by calling me names, such as *"fat batty, come here."* Being in school was also a problem because I was constantly teased and given the name *fat batty*. I was still in pain. The pain! From being subjected to this, I wanted a way out from the pain, by having a voice. But the pain became chronic, and I began to feel sensitive. All I wanted was for someone to value me for how I looked—with my African backside—to be loved, respected, and appreciated, and not to be seen as a weak person.

Creating my fish bowl environment was a place for me to try to let go of my pain. In addition, growing up as a child in a Christian faith, almost every Sunday, in church, I would hear the same saying, which went like this: "…..ask, and it shall be given; knock, and the door will open…." It's like when you are reading a novel, and you are in that imaginary world where the author takes you. All of a sudden, someone, or something, disturbs your imaginary world and, *snap, snap,* you are no longer there.

The place was an illusion. Not real! Knocking at the door for it to open was not happening when I was in the fish bowl. Being in that state of illusion, I had to tell myself to keep searching. I would say that my searching was for a person to share my entire life with, and not to be judged. This would be a man with similar attributes, such as being connected spiritually, emotionally, educationally, and financially, and having the drive to succeed beyond expectations.

Having said that, I felt I partly had that belonging through putting my trust into someone recently, rather than looking closely or deeply into my soul. Though searching all my life for the qualities named above, and being in the fish bowl, when he stopped corresponding, I was left by myself in the bowl, which later smashed into tiny pieces, with me gasping for breath. I was shattered and broken, and was unable to put the glass back together. It was painful. I learned a lesson from this, which was that things can be taken away from me in the flash of a moment. I know that many of us go through things like this. The fact is that when you invest in someone by giving them your *all*, and then they are no longer in your life, the feelings of loneliness, emptiness, betrayal, and vulnerability cramp your being. In the state that I find myself in now, every day, I accept ME for the person I am, and for the person I will become.

All the broken pieces from the gold fish bowl are for me—the extension of my greatness. Because I have accepted who I am, it is a crucial step for me to accept everything within the Universe. In doing this, my thoughts and feelings are that I can enjoy being happy with my own company and that of others. The fact that I had seen, and am looking at, the broken pieces from my fish bowl, showed me that I am awakened from the bowl that kept me *trapped* for years.

My greatness is now beginning. It's like a seed that has just been planted, and it is being given the correct environment to survive and grow into a tree. Life is the same: it flows through us, and we must accept ourselves as we are right now. However, it can be said that as a child growing up, most of our programming starts from parents, teachers, and our cultures, by them showing us how we should be, and not telling us that we are as great as we are. Accepting yourself is to live your life right at this moment, because there is no guarantee that you will be here tomorrow.

Whilst feeling poorly, and really looking deeply into my soul, I concluded that loads of people find it difficult to accept the joy that life is giving them; instead, they would rather be miserable. Why is this? They are programmed that way, so they create unhappiness in this way. They thrive by becoming miserable, and feeling very good about it. How sad is that?

Trust Yourself

From a very young age, I was told by my mum not to trust my father because he had never looked after me. For me, that was the beginning of *destroying* my mind. The only person I had then was my grandmother, who tried to teach me the fundamentals of building a relationship that was based on trust. It was difficult for me to trust myself because I saw what it had done to the relationship between my grandmother and me. She had to send me away from her to be with my mother in England. Soon after, she died. Who do I trust then?

No one! It was the beginning of me being afraid of making any decision, and being fearful that it will go wrong, at the age of eleven.

From my earliest teaching about not trusting my father, no other trust was possible, except that of my grandmother. But even then, it felt very artificial. It left me with unpleasant visions in my mind about trusting myself, and it made it strange and difficult. Surely, my parents were meant to be my first teachers, or should it be society? In that case, wherever they got their teaching does not allow them to trust themselves. For them, the biggest thing was to trust in their God, rather than knowing who they truly are. To be able to know who you are, and be an independent thinker, is not the *in thing*, but instead, an artificial thinker.

Neuroscientists carried out many investigations, and they concluded that we can't really trust our thoughts as well as our feelings to tell us what is going on inside of us. Maybe this might be the case because it's been said that the right side and the left side of the brain does not communicate effectively. Saying this, shows some confusion. As mentioned earlier, how I grew up has a lot to do with how I was taught, and the painful feelings I experienced.

To cope with any painful memories and feelings, which parents pass down to their offspring, we push them away and use tools for coping with these feelings. Food is a good example of this. In our society, we associate pleasure with eating red food such as meat, and pain with eating green food. Giving up something we love can be emotionally painful. We are driven to avoid pain but must seek pleasure. Sometimes an experience can put doubts in ourselves, so we don't trust our body, our thoughts, or our feelings to get through a situation.

One of my grandsons phoned me and appeared distressed. I would say he was in a *place* where he did not want to be. He was stressed about his relationship between him and his mum, to the point that I felt I wanted to reach out to him, especially when he said he did not know what to do to please her. Hearing this, I would say that he was in a tunnel and unable to see the light. Because of his limited experience, he might have thought that life was a *one-way street*, and not seeing it as a *fluid*, whereby when the liquid was thrown out, it would go all over the place. By it going everywhere, this will be where life should take him. I don't think he mastered the idea that it's up to him to find ways to make himself happy.

On the other hand, you have society telling you that to trust yourself is being selfish. It's at this point when your *inner voice* is telling you that you are not good enough, and you are beginning to doubt yourself. I would say my grandson was at that stage, whereby he was terrified of doing the wrong thing, and of making incorrect decisions and having to be responsible for the end results.

My grandson realised that by having a strong relationship with himself and others, he would know how to trust, even if a person tried to deceive him. He certainly knows that trust is a process that is valuable. In our quiet moments together, my grandson and I talked in depth to be mindful of what we think and feel, and to be aware that we can make mistakes and continue with our lives. We concluded that when we trust ourselves, it is the core of having good relationships.

Chapter 4

Meditation

"While physics and mathematics may tell us how the universe began, they are not much use in predicting human behaviour because there are far too many equations to solve. I'm no better than anyone else at understanding what makes people tick, particularly women."
Stephen Hawking

What Is Meditation?

Indeed, physics and mathematics may tell us how the universe began, but they are not much use in predicting human behaviour. In addition to this, many things in our lives are against our control. But we can take full responsibility to train our minds to empower our thinking. For me, it's the real *medicine* to our own personal sorrows, our anxieties, our fears, and our hatreds, together with a lot of confusion that controls our conditions.

I was living in a house with a person who would rather sit in the same position, day in and day out, watching programmes after programmes on the television, without even bothering to clean up the house or the room. I know that because, after a challenging time at work, the whole house is the same every day. *How often do I have to say that you have to start doing things in the house, and not just watch the dust and dirt getting the better of the whole house?* The answer is always the same. *I am not well.* When I would have enough, and would decide to clean the whole house, I would be told *"you have a bee in your bonnet."* Now you know why I must do what I must do. Over a period of time, the dirt started to accumulate, and the house became an unpleasant place for me to live. Of course, this is what he wanted. The air in the house was full of smoke from the cigarettes he started to smoke in the house. Basically, it was just a place of misery, chaos, and disorganisation.

Knowing what I just told you about my house, I can relate this to how my mind, body, and spirit operate. Misery, chaos, and disorganisation can be seen as unwanted things that we pile up in the form of negative energy as thoughts. The negative energy comes in many different forms, like the mass media, social media, socialising with various people, and looking deep within ourselves. In our society, a lot of us are too comfortable, because we have been taught to stay in our comfort zones rather than challenge our deepest fears and improve our situations, or be able to overcome any difficulties. Many of us are told, or shall I say conditioned, to believe that there is a quick way to fix any shortcomings by taking drugs. In this way, our behaviour remains the same, and the drugs will cure any illnesses.

I want to bring you back to the idea of the accumulation of dirt in my house, in terms of how our mind, body, and spirit work, without changing our attitude and lifestyle. In addition, with the dirt inside the body, we are now a living *dust bin*, with negative feelings and thoughts. This is why we need to get rid of them; otherwise, they are going to keep showing their ugly heads regularly, when you don't want to experience them. Albert Einstein summarised this as *"...insanity, doing the same thing over and over, and expecting a different result..."*

I must say that my understanding on getting rid of negative and emotional energies came when I was *down in the gutter,* and when I found the path of spirituality. In the past few months of having Bell's palsy, I have been meditating very early, daily, for an hour, as part of my morning routine. At first, it was a bit challenging because things were floating in my mind, and my energy was following them. Because of this, I knew my mind was not on healing my body. Just like when you are getting rid of all the mess in your house, which takes a while to clear and clean out the rubbish, it's in a similar way to get rid of the negative and emotion energy in our minds. It will take discipline and time to see the mess being cleared and cleaned out.

Saying this, I had to focus on my meditation to get the results I wanted. The regularity of carrying out my meditation became apparent. I noticed that once I acknowledged any distractions entering my mind, I had to let go of each one. Although there are many thoughts about the idea as to whether meditation is an African practice, it is certainly spiritual. It assists us to slow down, to be silent, and to become still, in preparation to become aware of our inner self, to create a balance of the physical and spiritual realm. It is the time to contact our mind, body and spirit. If we look closely at the root word, *medi*, as in *medicine*, it's to heal; therefore, meditation is a great source, where all true healing takes place.

When I meditate, the feeling of my whole body talking with me is a great sensation. Being self-aware in this way, I become more conscious of my thoughts, the ways my feelings are guiding me and, at the same time, focusing my attention on what I want in my life.

Mind, Body, And Soul

I now conclude that I am gravitating to things and places that are more peaceful and quiet than before I had Bell's palsy. The reason for me feeling this way is due to the fact that my facial nerve feeds a very small bone within the inner ear, which regulates any loud, sharp sounds. When my bone in the inner ear was being affected, every loud or low sound was received as a high shriek.

I had to move quickly from some people because the sounds were going through my left ear as if I was being stabbed by a sharp knife. To partly overcome this, I plugged my ear with cotton wool. Constantly, I wore a woollen hat that covered my ears. I still cover my ears while indoors but no longer plug my ears. The other thing that was soothing was to use a natural rose and lavender bath and body oil to massage my left side of my face. The oil helped to loosen any tightened facial muscles. I will never stop using the oil, and I will continue talking to my face at the same time, to encourage the muscles to move again, which is stimulating. It is also helping my face and my whole body to heal.

The reason why I am saying this is because the body, mind, and soul work as a system of energy. Working closely together, I know our mind, body, and soul keeps the energy flowing throughout our body. The energy flow can be disrupted according to our emotional state, such as being unwell, sad, or disconnected to our inner soul. To have a good energy flow, we must be in alignment by experiencing happiness in everything we do, and to treat our body and others with respect.

I want us to have a look at the mind. Les Brown, a motivational speaker, advised us that *"someone's opinion of you does not have to become your reality "* In view of this, we must have courage to examine that person's assumptions. We also need to be able to understand and work with our mind intuitively, disregarding any subtle destructions, and learn the skills to cultivate our inner strengths to trust our mind. I agree with Les Brown, because many of us fall into the hands of professionals, like teachers.

When I was in my first year of senior school, one of my teachers told me that I was only good with my hands, rather than using my brain; therefore, I should become a seamstress Because she was my teacher, I thought her opinion was correct. Who would argue with her, being my age? I did not become a seamstress. I am a qualified teacher, with three degrees. I learned to appreciate uncertainty through listening very carefully, without being prey to a person's opinion of who I am and what I will become. I am going to call it my conscious mind, because it's responsible for our thought processes, such as feelings, memories, and emotions, and how to interpret what we see.

Let us now look at the body. According to Dr. Sebi, a herbalist, *"the body is electric."* In that case, we are light beings. Where there is electricity, there must be light. We are constantly absorbing energy from the environment, as well as from the food we consume. Resulting from this, our body utilises the sources of energy to power each cell. Whilst carrying this out, the cells measure the level of electrical current that maintains the structure and function of our life. Therefore, the more electricity a person has, the more they are enlightened. This leads nicely into the soul.

For many years, I have been seeking to find that still, quiet place that some people talked about. I searched for the space of inner peace within me. It's that place where I would like to be enlightened through the flow of energy. Thinking this way is where I would see the soul as the *self*, the "I" that cradles the body and works through it. Being without a soul is like an invisible person inside a garment. Therefore, having a soul, the body needs life—being able to see and hear. With a soul, the body acquires the ability to think and have rational debates, and to develop personality and identity. It's the inner-self, our set of morals, values, and principles through the choices we make in life. An example of this is if a person knows that their value is to achieve and become successful in a business, then they should go for it. Indeed, you would expect that person to be striving towards it.

The soul is the spiritual reflection of your individuality as a person. It's the things that I honour that uplift me. It's a place where the energy is vibrating, which is in tune with my mind, my body, my soul, my ancestors and the Universe.

What Is The Spirit?

I want us to look at a possible definition of the word, *spirit*. The spirit is a non-physical part of a person, which is the *core* of emotions and the character. It is the *oneness* that is within and without. Being *within* is the part that creates a sense of peace, tranquillity, and balance, working alongside to understand nature. These develop the whole part of the person. Life itself is the whole part. There are many ways in which we need to work in unity to understand and support how life evolves. The idea of *without,* means to be connected with all forms of life in nature, and the relationship to the whole universe, together with the cosmic laws above the earth. The non–physical part of the person relies on their internal universe as their steps to carry them through life's journey, where the connections will take place.

Before I continue, spirit, in this discussion, is not about religion. I would like to stress that it's the interaction a person has with the Universe; therefore, religion can be seen as a *tool* or a set of 'rules' needed to understand the spirit, and to respect the energy around them, to be fully aware of the spirit. I agree with Martin Luther King Jr., when he said, *"Every man lives in two realms: the internal and the external."* Therefore, you can't have one without the other. They affect our thoughts with actions as well as behaviour. Basically, it's to do with matter, movements of the energy, and how they work together. The way we know the fundamental principles of how they work is through teaching and learning the rules of metaphors, like when the rain falls, it represents change that transforms life. Other fundamental principles are celebrations that involve listening to music, as well as dancing to certain ceremonies .

For ancient Africans, the fundamental principles required the involvement of studying mathematics, mastering science to understand cosmology, and natural medicine in order to apply the knowledge to the community where you live. The ancient Africans told us that we need to know the principles that govern the relationships between a person and nature, so that it's not just scientific but spiritual too. With this in mind, the knowledge of oneness is your reality, and being conscious of the present moment in time, of which we are guided by our ancestors, and the ways, things, or patterns in nature.

To be connected with your own spirit is when you know you are free of the past: when you don't have any issues, or even flashbacks, and your heart is free of the material world; you are not over-proving yourself but carrying out what you feel or know is correct for you, despite what others are saying about you. You know that your inner thoughts and energy are guiding you to carry out actions that will give you and others an abundance of great feelings, with a purpose. Being guided is the ability to connect and heal with the Creator as your power. Being guided and connected brings peace, tranquillity, happiness, freedom, and fulfilment, because you are no longer in conflict with the external complex realm of your mind and body. You are in the powerful *light source* of your spirit, to strengthen your growth through the journey and experiences of life.

How To Stay Focused

When I was growing up, especially in my teens, and to a larger extent, as an adult, at times, I found it challenging to stay focused.

Meditation

Maybe I was thinking in the wrong direction, which can be seen as mixed frequencies of consciousness and unbalance in my body, and therefore not being focused. Because, on my journey, I picked up lots of people's unwanted feelings, the idea of life being challenging for me was to stay focused. To stay focused, I would need to be in line with my body, and to know who I am, why I am here, and what is most important to me—consciously vibrating to stay focused. Having followed my inner thoughts, together with nature, I would be giving myself permission to be empowered and in a blissful body. In this case, one becomes wiser. There is a saying: Love thyself. So know who you are, and value it to stay focused.

If we go back to what I was saying in the few sentences of the first paragraph, there were, and still are, a lot of distractions around me to keep me from staying focused. Walking along the road, there were lots of noises, like people shouting and talking in their groups, or children crying, or other things in nature, such as birds tweeting, or the noise of traffic and trains. On many billboards, I saw businesses marketing their products, and the list goes on. If we cannot stay focused, then lots of us will not be productive to achieve tasks for the day. Rather than striving to go forward the way we want, we would be going backwards, whether focusing on relationships, hobbies, your business, or being in a classroom. It is crucial to stay focused so that we will get the results needed for the tasks. Staying focused is also crucial for happiness.

With your full attention on a given task, then your mind and your thoughts will be focused. In view of this, the given task would not be productive if you were texting, on the internet, or trying to talk to your business partner on Skype, or cooking food, and so on. Multitasking like this will certainly make you miserable. I often tell myself that during ancient times, people had many distractions. To receive our greatness, how do we stay focused in our lives? In our daily lives, we cannot have stress or tension, because this will further block us from being in tune with ourselves at that moment of time.

However, if we focus our attention on things that are challenging, then things would get more and more challenging. Instead, we must stay focused on drawing strength from the Creator, to enhance ourselves and get stronger. By doing that, the things that were challenging are no longer that huge steep mountain to climb, because the strength within will be greater than the challenge you are going through. In saying this, I have known what it's like to move through nasty challenges, from a very, very young age. I grew up in an abusive home, in every way you can imagine. I was abused emotionally, verbally, and sexually; and because of this, I know what it's like to break through the past, and to overcome the nasty challenges. Being in an abusive environment damaged my self-worth for years and years. These were the people I looked to as authority figures, to protect, support, and encourage me, and to raise me, at least into my teens. Because of the abuse I encountered, I really know what nasty challenges are, and they shouldn't stop the impossible from becoming the possible. Tossing, turning, and being in turmoil deep within, I somehow drew strength from a place that was much bigger than who I was. It was a place deep, deep within my soul. My break away started with what I needed to do in order to solve my problems on how I was being treated.

Staying focused is to unify ourselves, to avoid being distracted from our morality and values, so that we remain true to who we are. We can then value the teaching and learning, the spirituality and higher consciousness, and living, and the presence of the Universe, which you cannot describe. The Universe, at this point, is like a spiritual mystery that is beyond being put into certain groups. In this case, the teaching and learning is based on how to focus your attention on the object, how to be in stillness, and how to avoid being a victim, and to be vigilant and to have gratitude. To carry these through, we have to release ourselves from being locked up. Instead, we must remind our inner self on a regular basis. It might be working with nature, by having a photograph of an animal, a tree, or a bird. With this, it will bring you back, to stay focused on your purpose, because we can be easily distracted, and some people will do anything to take your mind off your intention. It's a bit like when a spider spans its web and is waiting for its prey to land on it, and the vibration on the web will attract the spider. To be distracted, therefore, is about falling into the trap. So, we have to find our way, through planning, to master the mind for it to stay focused, because sometimes, when you fall like the prey in the spider's web, you might not be able to get back up. Without being focused, you are not being true to yourself in a spiritual way. You must open the door, and allow the spirit in, to be authentic.

Opening Your Third Eye

I was always curious about this small organ. Like me, I know that many people have been fascinated about the realm of nature that might be beyond, or the reality of it. The fascination comes from what we cannot see or from which is a measurable universe. Many of us believe that something lies beyond our physical world, and that there is a way in which we can break through it and the spiritual realm. Indeed, there is a way that we can use our senses to view the unobservable, touch the untouchable, and hear things that we are unable to hear. This is our *third eye*. It's a part of our sensory organs, which is located between our brows, in the middle of the forehead. Sometimes it is referred to as the *mind's eye,* or the *inner eye*.

During my research, and from talking with people, I was shown similar things that highlighted the idea, where ancient people would describe the third eye (pineal gland) as being like an open door into higher intuition and knowledge. Another way of understanding the third eye is to imagine it as the *seed of the soul,* which is the things we give our soul to grow so that the outer shell can open. It symbolises a state of being aware of your *inner self*, through which the world can be seen in an extraordinary way. You will be able to see a wide range of different levels, together with dimensions and new things. Utilizing my third eye enabled me to have a greater control over my feelings and hearing. It's as if I was powerful whilst going through my journey.

Let us look at the pineal gland for a moment. As I mentioned earlier, it's located in the middle of the forehead, deep in the centre of the brain, and is dictated by light. It is very tiny and looks like a pine cone; hence, the name, *pineal*. The colour is reddish-grey. The pineal gland secretes a hormone called melatonin, which is a powerful antioxidant that is responsible for our sleep and wake patterns. It gets rid of free radicals, and it keeps us young looking. Melatonin secretion is low during the daylight but high during the dark, which can influence our reaction regarding the length of day versus the length of night. Certainly, it can affect our sleep patterns, especially if we carry out night shift work. Philosophers and other scholars believe that the pineal gland's full function is a bit of a mystery, whilst research suggests that we are getting closer to understanding the mystery of the pineal gland.

Ancient civilisations, such as the Egyptians, recognised it as the principal seat of the soul, and the place in which all our thoughts (intuitions) are formed. Many of us could say that we have had *a burning gut feeling*. For me, I think that the third eye governs our thoughts, and we have to be in readiness to receive new levels of knowledge and skills. This is where the idea of opening your third eye comes to reality. Our thoughts, ideas, and stories have to be reprogrammed, to become conscious, and to reinvent ourselves to change our reality. Being very sick with Bell's palsy, I had to reprogram myself by looking deep into the seat of my soul. I was running out of fuel because I had taken on far too many things in a day. I had to work and look after my family. I was like a headless chicken. Sometimes I couldn't eat my lunch. At times, I was so exhausted that I couldn't sleep. I was living without taking a breath. This is a form of conditioning, and I fell into the *trap*. I know many people were in the same situation as me, and some are still there right now. I had fears and doubts because I needed to work to seek security. And it was that emotion that I attached to money. Of course, this is a very low vibrational state, which I know many of you are in, even whilst I am typing these words.

My grandmother was full of some great sayings, like *"out of many difficulties, you will grow miracles."* Being on my consciousness journey, she was telling me that I need to make my present situation the best it can be, and to avoid any external forces that influenced my thoughts and feelings. It's like an alchemist type of consciousness hero, whereby the individual makes the worst situation the best, by transforming the negative energy into positive. Therefore, by opening my third eye, it gives me the freedom to think clearly, with clarity.

I need to let you know that some scientists noted that we see less than 1% of all wavelengths of light that exists, and we hear less than 1%. Does that mean we shouldn't bother to open the third eye? Because the third eye is like an organ in the mind, surely it can work collaboratively with our other senses to make it even more powerful. We can train it to be more refined and accurate, so that we can see the other 99% of light, and the other 99% of what we hear. With this in mind, using our intuition, we will be more aware of things that are not necessary. At a very young age, my grandmother was great at this. She would say that I must read what people are saying to me, in order to feel and see their souls.

Thinking about the ways my grandmother's thoughts worked at the time was a bit like being in someone else's shoes, whereby you are feeling their emotions. I didn't understand this, but looking back, she was guiding me to open my third eye, and to feel my surroundings. By doing this, my grandmother wanted me to use my energies, together with my inner soul, to further work with them. Now, I can use my knowledge and skills gained, to see or predict events that are not necessarily physical. Being able to do this, I know the difference between a fact or an opinion, and the interpretation of my third eye. Unfortunately, not everyone sees the same things; therefore, it would be difficult to share our perception with another person. Due to our unique qualities as individuals, we use different lenses to see the world, from various points of view. On the other hand, we have things in common, because everything that exists around us is up for questioning. Why is this? We can see that our world is changing at a vast rate; therefore, we need to ask questions about it. Are we being told lies about our existence?

Healing Through Visualisation

As a young girl growing up, I would hear this saying: A picture is worth a thousand words. I didn't understand it then, but the older I got, the more I valued the significance of it. For me, it's a form of visualisation that helps to foster healing. When shown a creative object, like a picture, or listening to calming music, we analyse it, then critically evaluate how that creative object or sound makes you feel. In doing these tasks, the artist has invited you to travel with him/her. During your travels, you are being guided to relax the mind and body connection. This allows the body to meditate. Whilst in the form of visualisation meditation, the picture we are imagining sends rays of light that touch our body. Doing this, you go deeper and deeper into your inner soul, which creates a space that can be opened so that visualisation can start to take place. Going through this balanced state, you get the feelings of calmness, wonderment, contentment, safety, and healing.

In the light of this, I want you to know that whilst being very sick with Bell's palsy, I used imagery a lot to help with my healing process. I would listen to soothing music that often depicted nature, such as birds chirping, with the sound of rain in the background. For me, this was a way of calling upon my innate healing powers, which stimulated the immune system. You might be saying that it's through my surroundings that this kind of healing is taking place.

My Grandma Aunty Jenny would tell me that we become what we think. Yes, she is correct! Indeed, I know our bodies react to how and what we think. Our thinking affects the glands of the endocrine system. They communicate between the brain and the body; therefore, when we have negative thoughts, they negatively affect the working of our body. Whatever thoughts you have, the hormones from the endocrine system are activated by every cell in your body.

In healing the body, I must say that visualisation in a repetitive way allows access to the mind, body, and soul, for it to be wholesome. Therefore, the mind, body, and soul works as a system to further enhance the healing process of the body, on a physical and spiritual level. An example of the mind, body, and soul, working as a system, is when we are physically hurt. This emotion generates a feeling, which turns into a physical sensation. We must think positively because it's crucial to the production of positive results. Thinking negatively and emotionally can lower the immune system. To be in a great state of mind, we must have positive thoughts and emotions; they activate the immune system to have an abundance of health and energy. I want to turn now to grounding, and how it affects our soul in the body.

Grounding

I would like to start off by looking at the word, *grounding*. Grounding is a spiritual term, which is referring to the core of the soul. This is also connected with Mother Nature.

As a very young girl, growing up in Jamaica, where there is an abundance of green lands, my Grandma Aunty Jenny would ask me to play in the *yard,* without my shoes. Of course, I had to go along with what she had said, without questioning her. Protecting me from taking on people's emotions, and from my surroundings, she would make sure that I was not exposed to these. She was making sure that I had a very strong connection with the spirit of Mother Earth. Despite what was going on around me, Grandma Aunty Jenny wanted me to stay balanced and aligned with my higher self.

What if you are not grounded? Being ungrounded is like a dandelion, and seeds are being blown by the wind because they are off balance. Sometimes, when you are not grounded, it is not a terrible thing. But it can be a problem if you are not grounded, because you will not be in control with your emotions, or your mental and your physical body. Therefore, you would not be able to ground yourself spiritually. Having said that, when you are grounded, it's like a massive tree, whereby any natural phenomena, such as the wind, will not influence you. Instead, whatever happens in the environment would not affect you, because you are at peace and more balanced.

I want to highlight an example of when you are grounded, and how you can respond in a way that is aligned with your highest self. If you are waiting at the bus stop, and someone accidentally steps on your toes, but you are grounded and balanced with your higher self, you would look past it, even if the person did not apologise. However, if you are ungrounded, your thoughts would be reflecting on an event that happened in the past, and which caused distress, and at that point, you may shout at the person who stepped on your toes, asking them to watch where they are going. In doing this, you are reacting to the situation, and using your energy of *not focusing* on the person. Clearly, it shows that you were also not focusing on what was happening at that specific moment in time.

In addition, when you're feeling any discomfort within your body, it can be difficult to be grounded, as I outlined above. Because of the tumultuous times, we must do our best to keep our body grounded. Having said that, it can be challenging to stay grounded when you are feeling sick; hence, you become emotionally vulnerable.

To overcome this, you will need to remember that when you are grounded, you naturally feel peaceful and balanced in the present moment. You will need to embrace the emotions and view it as energies travelling through your body. At the same time, avoid focusing on the emotions, because if you give them attention, they will grow and become intense. But when you allow the feelings, they will eventually disappear, once at the highest peak. At this point, you will be back again to ground yourself, because the emotions run their course. Being in this state of mind, you become blissful and peaceful, with a sense of alignment and balance in the body.

Chapter 5

Beyond Who You Are

"The answer is, who you are cannot be defined through thinking or mental labels or definitions, because it's beyond that. It is the very sense of being, or presence, that is there when you become conscious of the present moment. In essence, you and what we call the present moment are, at the deepest level, one."
Eckhart Tolle

Stop Holding Onto The Past

There is a saying: It is not what happens in one's life that matters, but it is the meaning one puts on what happens that matters. We are all individuals, with unique qualities. Learning from your mistakes does not mean you need to stop holding onto the past, but it's the meaning we put on it.

We are bombarded with lots of advice as to how to live our lives. I am sure you have heard things, such as to avoid looking back but to learn from any mistakes you made. You should never repeat them; however, if you find yourself in similar situations, then don't sit around worrying about them, but move on. Having said that, we will always think about our past; therefore, we cannot completely escape. Whatever is floating about in our thoughts, we must find strategies to avoid dwelling too much on the past.

As we embrace the idea of letting go of the past, it does not necessarily mean you totally forget about your unwanted thoughts, and leave them where they should be. You can turn them into wanted thoughts. Unfortunately, most of us are not taught to explain our feelings. Because of this, we have problems expressing our inner experience, and when we're not in touch, it's difficult to master this in a productive way. To be in a mind-set where you can identify how to hold on, or to let go of the past, is incredibly essential for having an abundance of health. You feel energetic. I would like to give my personal experience of this.

I met a man for whom I had deep feelings, and he said he felt the same. Whilst getting to know each other, after a year, we decided it was time to know more about our aspirations, goals, and ambitions, rather than texting or having the occasional phone call. Upon meeting him, and knowing a bit more about each other, he told me he was terrified of dogs, and showed me a mark on his foot where he was bitten. My heart went out to him, and I was feeling the pain that he had felt at the time. You might say, I was showing my emotions. Yes! As I was at his house, and about to go home, there was a dog by his doorway. Immediately, he closed the door, saying he knew the dog might have been there but did not want to tell me about it. According to him, he was protecting me. I appreciated his concern. But then, when we sat down to discuss ways to prevent the dog from being parked at his doorstep, I chuckled a bit, because I felt it was pathetic that people could leave the dog next to his door. Between him and me, we managed to report the fact that the dog was left unattended in that way. I told him it could have attacked him if he was unaware that it was left there, but he was not having it. He got very upset. He didn't want to talk to me, or even look at me. What do you do in a situation like this? With his behaviour, I was emotionally hurt. At that time, I was concentrating on the teaching I had from my grandma, which was to welcome his disappointment and to see it as a way to prepare myself emotionally and mentally, and to be ready for surprises that I did not necessarily want. With him being upset, I acted calmly, and was dignified, which enabled me to think clearly.

No matter how emotionally prepared a person might be, occasionally you can end up losing who you are, especially if you are holding onto the past. That's what being human is. Showing emotions, such as the one I shared above, can be messy, as well as leaving room for opportunities to cultivate compassion. This takes us nicely onto turning the page to look at your true self. I shall share my childhood experience to highlight some significant moments.

What Is Your True Self?

To know your true self allows you to tap into the realm of the conscious mind. This is where we bring good thoughts into our mind, and remove any unnecessary thoughts, to make our thinking clear. Having said that, when you understand this, and know what your true self is in terms of who you should be, then your purpose will become bigger than what you are fearful of. This brings us neatly into the following saying: Knowing your true self is the beginning of all wisdom.

The Spiritual Journey with Bell's Palsy

I know that my Grandma Aunty Jenny, in her own beautiful way, was teaching me the most important skill: to know my true self. She was driving my mind to focus and sharpen my commitments, to be resilient, and to persevere with challenges, even when they were difficult. Doing this, she was strengthening my powers, with which, at times, I had to stay still, without any movement or talking. I thought she was treating me bad for no apparent reasons. Grandma Aunty Jenny taught me that worrying would get me nowhere in my life, especially if I was unable to change the situation. She was good at telling me to be prepared for any disappointments.

Reasoning with me was something that I tried to understand, but it was challenging. However, Grandma Aunty Jenny would tell me that being prepared, when a disappointment comes my way, would give me the chance to turn it into an opportunity. Although I was very young, most times, I knew what to do rather than to seek permission from significant members of my family or others around me. Because Grandma Aunty Jenny inspired me to have the mind-set that competes with the most important person, it had to be my true self. I had to put myself first on the priority list.

Since the first two days of having Bell's palsy, I had to retrain my mind-set in order to think differently. As Michael Jackson told us through his song: *"I'm starting with the man in the mirror; I am asking him to change his ways."* My mind was calm and quiet, because I started with me, my true self. It was then that Grandma Aunty Jenny was telling me to think about her teaching; so, by hearing her voice, I began to acknowledge what to do. Doing that, I was drawn closer to my own true self. It was then that I started to meditate daily, for an hour, followed by reading the works of inspirational speakers. This kick-start set me up for the entire day. It's my enjoyment, whereby I stay focused and strong for the whole day.

Affirmation

Come with me to look at what an affirmation is. An affirmation is a powerful statement that affirms something to be true. When you think about a statement, or you hear it or say it, then it becomes your reality. Therefore, you are being conscious and in control of your thoughts. Having said that, you are bringing the vibration of energy, and releasing that energy into the Universe. In essence, whatever we say, is an affirmation. It can either be positive or negative thoughts. With your thoughts going into the Universe, you are creating them, so any good ones that you have will allow you to take control of the bad ones that might want to take over. There is a saying that you might have heard, which goes like this: Be careful of what you think; because what you think, is what you get.

From growing up with my grandma, my affirmation was that having a good career opportunity, or good relationships with people, would never work out for me. Because I put these self-defeating ideas in my mind, it had left me being very critical. I refused to know that anything good would every happen to me. My perception was that everything would be wrong. Therefore, I created these situations, which were always right, because I wanted to see them.

When I started to realise the grooming that Grandma Aunty Jenny had given me, I started to consciously search spiritualism, and then my mind-set changed. My mind took on a different state, and the words that I would think of had taken on many meanings. By fine tuning this approach, things that I thought of and said, I would see them almost instantly. This was me working with the Universe, and it responding to the signal that I sent through my emotions. In saying this, my mind and emotions must be saying the same thing. It must be said, at this point, that it took me a very long time to know what was happening to me.

In terms of me having a close relationship with a man, the signals I was sending was to have a *good-looking* man. Looking back now, I was very vague; therefore, it didn't matter if he was not smart, or he was cheap, selfish, a liar, unfaithful, or egotistical. Despite these qualities, he had to be *good-looking*. Unfortunately, for me, that was the kind of relationship I got. Looking for the idea of a good-looking man, I would find things that were *wrong* with me. When looking at myself, I would say that I was too fat, with a big backside, and my nose was too broad. Having a good-looking man was a way for me to hide my faults, because he would accept me, and no one would notice any inadequacy that I created. Indeed, I met the *good-looking* man. He was too good-looking, and I got worried, because I wanted to know what was so great about me that he liked.

Once again, I told myself that it would never last. Each message I received from him, or from being in his presence, I tried my hardest to accept that he wanted me for who I was, and that he appreciated my qualities. My struggle was very painful, which made me unhappy, even though it was in my thoughts. To him, it didn't seem to cause any problems. Telling myself that he was for me, allowed me to accept the relationship, although I was not happy. But having that *good-looking* man in my life made me accept him, because he wanted me, even though he had many flaws. I had to convince myself to accept them, because he was *good-looking*.

Being well into the relationship, I realised that things were not as they were, so I took it upon myself to express my feelings. When I asked him why he was no longer sleeping in our bed with me, he tried to smile it off, but I continued. To work on this, I gave him some ways that we could solve the problem, but he looked right through me, as if I was talking nonsense. With his inquisitive look, I asked if I had said something misleading. It was then that he replied by saying, "What makes you think that I want to be in the same bed as you?" He went on to criticise my big nose, and the fact that my backside was huge, and he asked, "When did you last look at yourself in the mirror?" This man showed me all those negative things, and I learned to believe them as the truth.

Our thoughts, together with what we say aloud, are crucial, because we may not realise that we are creating them, whilst repeating them over and over. In this way, we certainly will see them come true, but we do not recognise those things we asked for as becoming a *self-fulfilling prophecy*. Sometimes, when it manifests itself, we feel hurt, frustrated, betrayed, and in denial, because of how they showed up in our lives. Our thinking and speaking are energy we use to focus our mind. Therefore, we must be aware of what we are putting out in the Universe. In saying that, your thoughts about your reality create your experience of that reality, through speaking the words. So, affirmations are ways to create emotions in a positive way, so we can create all that we want. They must be specific, and convincing, because words have power. Now, I want you to walk with me and take a moment for reflection.

A Moment For Reflection

When you are being reflective, you are showing careful consideration about something. Many of us have created a crisis, one way or another, in our lives. Why? The crisis that I created was finance. Lots of you would agree with this. My heart used to miss a beat when I would see piles of letters being dropped through the letter box onto my carpet. Every morning, I would be thinking to myself that an official would be coming to turn off the electricity or the gas, or to re-possess an item.

As a young child, I was never taught the value of saving money, or to budget. My immediate family struggled financially. Once they had money, it would go as quickly as when they received it. Because of this, I thought I didn't have money to save; therefore, there was no need to save. I never saved. There was a saying from a few adults in my family: Money is the root of all evil. Seeing how my family and I lived hand-to-mouth, I grew curious and intrigued. Much of my spare time was spent reflecting, whilst thinking of the statement those adults said, about money being *evil*. Maybe that was the reason they did not teach in schools how money can work for you. Who wants to learn about evil? It was then that I began thinking, for long periods of time, of all the things I would do when I had lots of money.

At long last, I had money. Not having so much, I spent it on all sorts of things. Because I had never had it, I was making up for what I did not have. The financial crisis happened, and affected me to the extent that I didn't know what to do. Most of the money I had was gone. My children needed to eat, and I had to pay bills. This was the same for many of my friends, and I believed other people were in financial crisis like me. Some were on Social Security, from the government, for financial support. We were in a sticky situation. My Grandma Aunty Jenny would often tell me that people live their lives by being fearful and being greedy. She was correct! These two ideas are feelings we get, especially being without money. A lot of us become fearful; hence, most people believe that we have to work much harder than before. The moment the money is in our hand, we become greedy, and the mind will be imagining all the things we want. Of course, we then start spending. I believe my grandma was warning me to be careful, to avoid being overindulged, and to think in a logical way.

Whilst reflecting on these, I went for a walk, and I saw the following in a newspaper: "The financial crisis happened because banks were able to create too much money, too quickly, and used it to push up house prices and speculate on financial markets."

Reading this, my attitude toward spending changed quickly, and I followed up on what my Grandma Aunty Jenny would always tell me to believe: Whatever happens, you can get what you want, but you need to believe you can get it. As mentioned before, our thoughts are very powerful, so we can create a mind-set to turn them into making whatever we want.

How To Accept Change

Life is such a wonderful gift. With this gift of life, it's unpredictable. Therefore, life is not permanent, which means that everything changes. In a flash of light, things can happen that will transform you as an individual. In this case, who you were and what you have become can impact your life. Because of the changes that impacted your life, you need to embrace it and accept whatever comes to you. It might be that you see yourself as ordinary. That's fine, because it's the first step towards becoming extraordinary. Therefore, this is one way to develop the ability of looking into yourself, through positive thinking, instead of negative, which is defiant.

To accept changes in our lives brings a lot of different challenges. When my uncle died a few years ago, it was difficult for me to accept, because we had a close bond. Another change I had to accept was when I was sick with Bell's palsy due to the viral infection in my ear. It was challenging for me to accept or to embrace the suffering that my whole body was going through. Although I had to deal with it, a part of me was thinking that such a thing as that should have never happened. So, being through what had taken place in my body, my mind changed to thinking that everyone must start by cultivating acceptance in all areas of their lives. Doing this, we will be more able to cope with whatever crises come to us; therefore, we will be more able to cope with the different challenges.

Of course, by having a mind-set that allows us to look to the future and be prepared to cope with crises, we will be more willing to accept the change rather than resisting it. At one point, I felt as though I was resisting the viral infection and the terrible pain that my body was going through, I had a lot of turbulence in my mind. With such feelings, I had to eventually realise that there was no option but to accept the choice, and continue with my life, as well as constantly talking to myself and being positive. In doing these things, my mind started to flow steadily, instead of feeling the turbulence in it. I was accepting changes within my body—my Grandma Aunty Jenny would tell me to appreciate what is now happening, by being grateful, when my life was *bitter*—therefore, saying thanks, and then growing with it.

She was so correct. With her teaching and guidance, a couple of years ago, I had really learnt how to fully understand the power of acceptance. Someone came into my life, and we used to text and have the occasional phone call, which seemed to be his way to communicate. I went with it. It was like a testing ground, which I was happy with, despite being very nervous to meet someone, after about 10 years without any commitment with a man.

It was over a year before we started to spend quality time together to get to know each other. A few months later, he appeared to be very busy, and he told me he was working and unable to look after himself. Our relationship started to be stagnated; although I asked questions, he was reluctant to answer them. With his behaviour, and mine, I concluded that I had no option but to accept whatever his problems were, and to continue with how I was before meeting him, to move my life to its next level.

What have I learnt? Well, it was extremely difficult for me. With my mind-set and the closeness I had with my grandma, and listening to her talking to me, I found the strength and an inner peace to accept it, instead of trying to change the situation, which was beyond my control. Acceptance is an emotional feeling, which is a choice, and can be extremely deep. In a way, it's a bit like me protecting myself, with a shield, from getting hurt. Acceptance can move from a feeling of happiness to being very happy within one's soul. Now, I want you to walk with me, to look at being in harmony with nature.

Being In Harmony With Nature

The mind is a powerful *tool,* which allows us to be aware of the world through our thinking, judgement, perception, and consciousness. It's like a road. In this case, when we walk along the road, we perceive various things, such as plants, animals, and trees. With these things, we, as humans, need them in nature to exist, because we are all interconnected in what I would say is the web of life. Because of the web of life, it is crucial to create a balance to use the natural resources in a similar way to other species. Saying this, we must be careful to avoid exploiting our natural resources, because it will create a *knock-on effect*, whereby other generations might not survive.

To achieve a balance, society must be equal. It needs to be maintained and be sustainable through social development and having a sufficient economy. The interconnection we have with nature, therefore, must be a harmonious one, which means that when we are consuming natural resources, it must be at a similar pace in line with what nature generates. Earlier, I mentioned the idea relating to walking along the road and looking at the ecosystems during your journey. We can see that there are many things in our environment that are affecting the depletion of our natural resources. For example, with the advancement of technology, it's giving rise to another problem. Children are now hooked on the internet and playing games. Because of this, their physical activities and exercises are becoming considerably less. The same health problems are amongst adults, and we are seeing that many of us are suffering from all sorts of diseases. Also, the usage of fertilisers is affecting the soil, and as a result, it's losing its natural fertility. Consequently, some varieties of plants became extinct.

Being in harmony with nature is essential for both Earth and our health, together with the well-being of humanity. I am not saying the development of technology is not a good thing; it should not have any detrimental effect on the present and the future generations.

Depleted Soils

For many years now, people have been told that the poor-quality soil is not a problem, but then it relied heavily on synthetic fertiliser products. These fertilizers kill a large amount of the naturally occurring tiny organisms. The micro-organisms bacteria that were present would break down the natural organic substance into plant nutrients. As a result, they would further help with the conversion of nitrogen, an essential nutrient for plant growth. Another useful soil bacteria are the ones that make sure bugs and other parasites are not out of control.

With depleted soil, we can see nutritional deficiencies in fruit and vegetables. For example, they are being picked well before they are ready to be eaten. Many of the tomatoes that are non-organic are being made to look red by using certain chemicals, rather than the natural sunlight.

You might be thinking that it's the soil that is losing out on essential nutrients. No! Our health is affected too. Many oils that used to occur naturally in our food are not how they used to be. Some of them, like the omega oils, are said to lead to serious illnesses, such as heart disease and cancers. We don't get enough niacin because of the processed food we are taking in our body. Niacin is crucial for the digestion of food and to maintain a healthy nervous system. This nutrient can be found in foods such as dairy products and nuts.

Chapter 6

The Awakening

"What really matters is not whether we have problems, but how we go through them. We must keep going on to make it through whatever we are facing."
Rosa Parks

Self-Fulfilment

With Rosa Parks' statement above, the meaning is powerful in terms of how we go through our problems. Looking at the main cause of any illnesses or chronic conditions in our society, the overriding cause is a deep feeling of emptiness and meaninglessness. Definitely, it's "… how we go through them," and this is why "we must keep going…." For this reason, the self-fulfilment idea comes into fruition, which is so important.

Although self-fulfilment is solitude, it enables us to truly discover what will fulfil us, so that we can live a purposeful life, where the idea of *freedom* and *true happiness* is *strong*. I will touch on this in the next section. Not only does solitude help us develop self-fulfilment, which we all seek to find, this can be in a spiritual state during our journey of life. If you have fallen into the rut of life, and no longer feel like your true self, why not go for a holistic healing retreat to awaken your essential self. Go to my website, successwithbellspalsy.com, for more information.

Happiness

For the past few months, I find myself alone. One thing I always avoid is to be in solitude. Despite this, I feel as if I am no closer to happiness. However, while I agree that you can reach momentary appreciation and happiness, those brief moments are never deeply fulfilling for me. My Grandma Aunty Jenny told me on several occasions that happiness is when you are fulfilled. Therefore, it should not drain your energy. Instead, it must add more, and this is where happiness comes from outside things; because of this, it tends to disappear when the situation changes. If, shortly after your wedding, as a newly married couple, one of you has a serious accident, the pleasurable experience of being married will certainly disappear due to the serious accident that person had.

As a child, I knew my grandma was telling me that it's a state of the mind, because you can have everything in the world and still be miserable. Fulfilment is the key here for me, and this is what I seek. Once you have mastered the art of appreciating and consciously enjoying what you already have, whether or not it's an unpleasant thing you are going through, I would say it's an example of happiness, because the other things, such as pain, are insignificant.

I want you to come with me and have a look at joy. But before we do that, I am going to leave you with John Lennon's idea of what happiness is: *"When I was 5 years old, my mother always told me that happiness was the key to life. When I went to school, they asked me what I wanted to be when I grew up. I wrote down, happy. They told me I didn't understand the assignment, and I told them they didn't understand life."* This shows that happiness is external, and is based on your situations, events, people in your life, and your thoughts.

Joy

Joy is a spiritual quality that is internal. I watched my Grandma Aunty Jenny having a lot of joy, and I learnt from observing it. Her man ran off with her life's savings. She realised it when she had to pay for her unit in the Carnation Street market, in Jamaica. Because of this, she was forced to live a simple life, whereby she shared a single bed with four members of the family, to save money. My Grandma Aunty Jenny recycled many things, such as her clothes, and whenever she drank any drink from a bottle, that too was recycled. Most importantly, what she recycled best of all was her pain, which turned into joy.

From such betrayal, it was a privilege and an enigma to watch my magnificent grandma's life emerge with power. Rather than looking externally for another man to take away the ashes of betrayal, she had to rise above it. Rising above that relationship, she cultivated and embraced internal and deep abiding joy. As you can see, throughout my spiritual journey, I use her a lot as an example of a powerful woman, and of someone who put away greed and fear, and allowed balance into their higher self. For me, this is the joy of life. Now, I want you to look at the next section on ideas and realities.

Ideas And Realities

A possible meaning of an idea is *the thoughts that generate in the mind*, whereby reality is *the quality of being real*. From this, I would say the mind can create a world of illusion. When we change our thoughts, we change the idea, and then the experience is a different reality. In this case, our mind is a powerful *muscle*, which controls the thought process, and therefore allows the mind to be conscious of the world.

The mind selects the possibilities, and determines, by selecting which information to observe, and at the same time, knowing if it's real. To have an idea that things are real, we rely upon our senses to interpret the world. Objects in our world are examples of how we use the senses. Our hearing, our smell, our touch, and our taste are some of the senses the mind uses to tell us about how real objects are. Using our sight to observe the magnificent beauty of nature's patterns, sizes, etc. is a sense that informs us that it's not just an idea but real.

Accepting An Emotion

Being unstoppable, and knowing yourself, is accepting your emotion. Look closely at what I said. Now, think about it for a moment! Yes, yes, you are the awareness behind what you are thinking here, together with the emotion. In some ways, it might be difficult to describe an emotion because of the complexity of it. However, there are signs of emotions that we can observe, such as body language, which includes facial expressions, crying, tones of voice, rapid breathing, and restlessness.

The Awakening

Let us look at the idea of an emotion! It can be a deep feeling, like that of two people falling in love. Each of them might have a slightly different interpretation about their feelings. Therefore, emotions affect many areas of a person's life, and a person can affect various aspects of that emotion. A person's emotions can affect them physically, as much as their feelings and how they think. If a person were to avoid these, then they might not be true to themselves. As a result, the emotion can show up in a physical way, like having a serious illness, such as cancer. This is why we must *let go* of our feelings. Letting go will enable you to manage it, because I don't think you can control it.

Chapter 7

The Unquiet Mind

"Sometimes the heart sees what is invisible to the eye."
H. Jackson Brown Jr.

Worrying About Worrying

We all worry from time to time. It's a matter of not being able to get the mind to settle. Worrying about worrying can therefore get bigger, because you become anxious. Because of this, it can easily be directed inwards. In this case, you might be thinking about unnecessary things, like being burgled, or aging, or death which can become self-fulfilling if they are allowed to continue. Unrelenting worries can be paralyzing if you can't get negative thoughts out of your head. In view of this, they can sap your emotional energy and interfere with your daily life.

Worrying can even be helpful, if it spurs you to take action to solve the problem and make a logical decision. But it's crucial to clarify what the problem is. Once you realise this, then stay focused, and completely turn off those anxious thoughts so that you can regain control of your worried mind. In addition, you need to view whatever the problem is, as a challenge or an opportunity, which you will appreciate at the end of it. Thus, worrying is an automatic habit of your thoughts, in response to particular events. It's stimulated by something we are thinking of, which is then triggered automatically deep within. Worrying about worrying, is certainly not a natural state of our way of life, nor is it a good idea.

Sometimes I would worry about things, such as being late for an appointment, or I would avoid opening the brown envelope with my examination results because of the fear that my results would be unsatisfactory. Then, after a certain time, my worries start to decrease on their own. Because we are never taught how to face it, we must feel the fear and do it anyway. The result is that we show ourselves, despite the situation, that we can manage it. Go to my website, successwithbellspalsy.com, for more information on acceptance rather than control.

Keeping Worries To Yourself

As a young child growing up with Grandma Aunty Jenny, we always talked about many issues. I knew then that I was fortunate to have her. Going to school for me was problematic because I did not want her to leave me. Without minimizing my worries, she would tell me that lots of problems will go away. What she was telling me was that they were temporary and could be solved. Some days I would worry about things, like making myself look silly if I messed up the times tables, which we had to recite daily. To reassure me, and to offer her comfort, Grandma Aunty Jenny would say that some days will be better than others. Despite my worries, she was showing me how to keep my problems in perspective, which then lessened my worries. Because of this, she was giving me the tools to help build my strength and become resilient.

Keeping worries to ourselves might be challenging. Why do I say this? It's been noted that a large proportion of people suffer from anxiety disorders. This might be characterised by unnecessary worries, which can then lead to other physical symptoms. Surely, worrying is largely to do with how we process information in our brain. In this case, we naturally worry about how to solve a problem systematically, and then we think through each step logically.

Our fast paced, technological, and noisy world that we now live in has a vast impact on our lives. Therefore, the brain is overwhelmed with stimulations from various points, which also affects our behaviour. Ideas that over stimulate the brain can affect our decisions; and hence, we worry. Take time, every day, to experience a quiet moment, and be still, which can help with your worries.

Emotional Reactions

An emotional reaction tells us how to respond to life's experiences. It might be showing fear. Imagine, whilst shopping in the mall, someone offered you a snake to handle. In this case, you might show two conflicting emotions. For example, you might show excitement and fear. These two emotions enable you to observe them, so you are in the position to approach the snake with caution. Being fearful is the emotion, and your caution is the reaction towards the snake.

Instead of avoiding or suppressing your emotions, you can learn from them through turning to that experience. Open to the fear, and bring compassion towards it, rather than fighting it. If you put up a fight, you will strengthen it. Whilst doing this, you are accepting the emotion and observing its awareness, as well as the reaction it gives you. Saying this, now, I want you to take a walk with me and look at the ideas of values.

Your Values

It's fundamental to know that sometimes the heart sees what is invisible to the eye. In this case, we face tough decisions every day of our lives. So, your values demand the whole body.

My Grandma Aunty Jenny taught me some excellent values, such as being **truthful**, and according to her, some days would be naturally better than others. For her, this was the same as having my relationship with other people, which can get shaky at times, but staying devoted to a person through uncertain times can be the *rock* to grasp.

Another value that she taught me was to have **integrity.** This value defines my character and the ways in which I react, and how I respond to certain things that occur. **Respect** was the one that she would dwell on though, because I had to show how to think, together with how I believe. As an adult, I know that to show respect is also validating a person's dignity, and enhancing my own.

Most of these values are challenging to carry through because of the society in which I live. Despite challenges, I am open to changes, but my values taught by my grandma will never go away. Being a parent and a professional, my character, together with my peace of mind, are constantly tested. Developing my skills through practicing everyday as a child, I was determined and persistent, which paid off, because my words and actions were in balance with my values. If there was a mismatch in terms of my behaviour, then I would know that something was wrong. It would cause discomfort within my whole body.

Powerful Autopilot

"Sometimes the heart sees what is invisible to the eye." This statement is so lovely. I like the idea that the heart sees what the eye doesn't. With autopilot on, our eyes are not focusing on things, because we are mentally unaware.

Being on autopilot, for me, is like going to work every day, whilst carrying out the same routine, before setting out for work. At the same time, I am feeling overwhelmed with trying to get rid of long held grievances in a relationship. Because of this routine, it was making my choices, in whatever I carried out, challenging. Over time, it was becoming seemingly impossible to shift.

I would say, at this point, that my mind was clouded by thoughts and feelings, and I was preoccupied most of the time; hence, being on automatic pilot. With this, I did not reflect on my thoughts and feelings; instead of dismissing them, I allowed them to enter my mind.

Looking back at skills, my Grandma Aunty Jenny taught me mindfulness, which was to be tolerant when feeling discomfort or being distressed in any way. The stance that she took was for me to be *still*, and to observe my thoughts, and then slowly let go, without empowering them. Certainly, she was correct, because I was preparing myself to become free from being uncomfortable whilst facing a stressful situation. With this in mind, let us examine the idea of uncertainty.

Uncertainty

What I know is that our life has a lot of turning points. Knowing this, it comes as no surprise that we go through uncertainty, no matter what we do. Due to turning points in our life, unexpected events happen, which cause changes. Uncertainty is uncomfortable. Because of this, some people become reactive by what's going on around them. When your vibrations are leading you to someone you care for, and you are experiencing the worst that might happen, then you must remind yourself that no matter how the relationship works out, you certainly can learn to be true to yourself, and you can still be happy, regardless of the situation that lies in front of you.

Others will clearly avoid any situations that may have uncertain outcomes, so they set realistic visions or goals. People who carry this through give themselves enough time and discipline to achieve whatever they want. On the other hand, life would be boring if we did not have uncertainties. This brings us to look at transformation.

Chapter 8

Transformation

> *"You can't have a physical transformation until you have a spiritual transformation."*
> Cory Booker

What Is Transformation?

The word, *transformation*, can be a sudden change of character, or in appearance. Saying this, everyone goes through it in a natural way. This change can be seen as a process of your life being raised to a higher level, therefore amazing new things will be happening to you. Sometimes it can be painful, especially if you are going through an illness. In my case, during the process of going through the condition of Bell's palsy, I wanted to be alone. It is part of my spiritual journey for me to look deeply into my inner soul in order to find out about ME. My Grandma Aunty Jenny would tell me to sit back and take a deep breath, to fill my lungs, and then let go, and go with what is going on. Was this her way of showing me the process of transformation?

Gratitude

For me, gratitude is an emotional feeling in response to a choice being made. It might be that you choose to be either grateful or ungrateful, depending on the situation. Being with my grandma, we always showed each other an expression of gratitude, and I would say it creates a healing effect. It was a natural thing to show our appreciation for the smallest or biggest thing. A very crucial thing, like saying thank you, was something that Grandma Aunty Jenny cultivated in me, culturally and psychologically.

As highlighted earlier, that gratitude is an emotional feeling. It brings me to the state of how we now live our lives in this modern, technological world, without practicing gratitude. Being a primary school teacher, and teaching students on a daily basis, I see that they seem to have lost the essentials to be grateful, despite giving them the *tools*. Most adults also forget to show the importance of gratitude. If we take a look at all the distractions we encounter in our daily lives, perhaps they become too many to show things like compassion and generosity. When we, as adults, practice gratitude, together with encouraging children to do the same, then it will cultivate lives with a purpose.

Reality Versus Illusion

I shall start this section by saying our mind is a powerful tool, which governs everything, and what you can do with your mind is exceptional. In this case, our mind works alongside the senses; therefore, we perceive things as real, so we go along with them to get along. If we got hit by a car, and damaged an area in our body, we would feel pain and discomfort, and it would be difficult to say it's unreal. Despite this, some people would say it's an illusion. Thus, the mind creates an illusion.

Being in several yoga sessions, and having to focus my attention on an object whilst carrying out a particular pose, I was unaware of movements and sounds in my surrounding. It was as if I was creating my own world from a different viewpoint. I was. This shows that, at times, we are conscious of the world, but sometimes we are not. It's crucial to be conscious of how you see things because, if you are not, someone will certainly create them for you. Now, come and dive deep with me! I promise you, you will not drown.

Diving Deep

Diving deep is when you can learn to focus and to heal your inner soul so that you can strengthen the unlimited powers within. Your unlimited powers might have been lost due to the technological world we are now experiencing. The soul is powerful because it encompasses passion, intuition, emotions, and creativity, which are connected with the Creator. Regardless of your life's journey, you can dive deep into your inner soul to create a lifestyle that is meaningful, with a purpose.

Many of us will deny our inner most soul because of the changing world we are in, thus the vibration of the soul becomes imbalance. By diving deep into our feelings, we will connect to our soul, and at the same time, get rid of the repressed emotions, like anger, hurt, fear, and disappointment. Doing this is a great way to transform the soul, and to develop who you are.

Be Selfish

I am reminded every day to take care of myself. Does that mean I need to schedule some *me time*? In fact, having a strong grandma in my life from an early age, who showed me ways to be grounded, by putting myself first, has enabled me to get whatever I need. Being grounded at an early age taught me to focus on my mind, body, and soul, and to be authentic, despite how others perceived me.

I often give away a lot of my energy by serving people's needs and wants. Realising their vibration, I began to be selfish and focused more on myself, so that I could take much better care of ME. To stay focused and get what I want or need, I meditate a lot. I am mindful of my relationship with people, and I eat well and exercise frequently. Unapologetically, I would say, I am selfish.

Being selfish is a good thing. My grandma used to tell me that it's the best way to happiness. Now I know that when I seek happiness, I am helping others to be happy; because, as Dennis Brown reminds us in his song, "No man is an island." We are all significant in Mother Nature. We need each other.

Negative Visualisation

"Positive visualization helps you get what you want. Negative visualization helps you want what you get." Let us look at negative

visualisation from what this quote is highlighting. It might be that your thoughts are on something that is significant, but you imagine it had gone, such as being evicted from your house and living rough on the streets. This can apply to any situation in our lives, because everything is on loan, and can be taken from us at any time. Our health or a loved one can be taken away in a split second.

A close friend of mine once said, "I appreciate YOU." This was because I was apologetic for something he did. Was this a dummy run for something real to come? *Grandma Aunty Jenny* would tell me that I am the creator of my thoughts and can make anything happen, through visualisation. Because I was largely oblivious to her teaching, and I just wanted to play with my peers, I didn't know that she was preparing me to align my vibration.

Encouragement From Mother Earth

Mother Earth can be seen to represent an abstract quality, a goddess of fertility, and vegetation. In this case, all species have at their disposal a wealth of natural energies from Mother Earth, which can be used as useful healing tools. She talks to us, and we must listen.

Herbs provide a tangible sign of transformation and growth. They provide an endless source of supply that heals and energises our bodies. Because of their qualities, even the scents, whether touched or not, can affect our bodies. The calming Lavender is known to stimulate happiness and to promote good sleep.

The Spiritual Journey with Bell's Palsy

I can recall when I was going for a walk through the woodland with my grandma, during a strong wind. I was worried. Feeling my emotion, Grandma Aunty Jenny held me tight. With her holding me, I felt my breath was being strengthened by the wind. It was as if it had cleared my mind by telling me that we were both safe and must not be scared. Like mothers, the energy of the wind looks after the health of the offspring. Looking at this from another dimension, I would say it is physical and spiritual, with an emotional healing.

I must say *our health is our wealth*, and it's a crucial part of Mother Earth. She might not be able to fix many of our major health problems, due to the slow climate change, but we must play our part by looking after our health.

Chapter 9

Recovery

"If you're trying to achieve, there will be roadblocks. I've had them; everybody has had them. But obstacles don't have to stop you. If you run into a wall, don't turn around and give up. Figure out how to climb it, go through it, or work around it."
Michael Jordan

Temporary Weakness

Indeed, obstacles don't have to stop you. You can recover from Bell's palsy, because the condition that inflamed the inner ear, which causes damage to the facial nerve of one side of the face, is temporary. Because we are all different in our make-up, with a condition such as Bell's palsy, there is a wide variation, which makes it difficult to give a definite time of recovery. For me, I was told by many medical specialists to be patient, because the condition is temporary.

Whilst recovering, I noticed a few problems, like dryness in my eye, and a runny nose, especially when driving. I would say this was caused by the fumes from my car, which was irritating. The lesson I learnt here was to stay away from strong fume-like chemicals whilst recovering from Bell's palsy. In saying that, lots of developments were taking place in the affected side of my face. Experiencing these changes, with some little facial movements, I was told that the nerves were recovering.

The Onset

For some people, like me, the symptoms were very sudden, which was over night. Other people might develop it at a slow rate, over time, without noticing it. The onset can occur for a few days or months. Since recovery can be quick, with the body taking on a natural healing process, some people will sit back and wait for it to happen. Spontaneous recovery can take place, for the majority of people, within one to two weeks after the onset of the symptoms. Like me, I would say other people with Bell's palsy will make a good recovery within the first three months, but occasionally, a mild symptom, such as tightness in certain areas of the face, will occur. Others may not recover so quickly within the first three months, but will have persistent symptoms of weakness.

As soon as you are feeling unwell, it is crucial to visit your general practitioner (GP) so that they can investigate any medical problems that you might have. Doing this will certainly put your mind at rest, because you don't want any roadblocks to stop your daily progress. Therefore, an early diagnosis is important so that you will be given the correct advice.

Within 9 Months

Because Bell's palsy is a temporary condition, most people make a full recovery within 9 months. It can take even longer and, in a small number of cases, the facial weakness can last a lifetime. If your facial weakness is causing problems in terms of disempowerment, then surgery might be a possible treatment, but you need to discuss it with your general practitioner (GP). It is said that children who suffered with this condition make a full recovery.

Let's examine my recovery. During my recovery, I felt the nerves in my face doing all sorts of strange things. Maybe they were trying desperately to reach the muscles so that they could be balanced. Here are some examples:

- My left eye was closing and in balance with my right one.
- Although my smile was much better, it remained a bit weak.
- Rather than my face looking asymmetrical—meaning that both sides were uneven—with recovery, it is now symmetrical (similar parts are even), especially when I am relaxed. I would say the muscles are more toned and are not floppy.
- My left eye appeared to be smaller than the right one.
- At times, my left cheek felt tight and stiff.

It was weird to observe how some of my muscles moved together instead of separately. When I smiled, my left eye would close, which then affected my cheek. It would tighten the moment I raised my eyebrows.

As mentioned above, even with the nerves in my face doing all sorts of strange things, it was possible to restore more normal movement again, with specific and appropriate exercises and expressions. I want us to now have a look at some of the exercises that I was asked to carry out daily.

Exercise

As Michael Jordan suggested, "...If you run into a wall, don't turn around and give up. Figure out how to climb it, go through it..."

This is so true! Because my facial muscles on my affected side were doing all sorts of unwanted movements, they had to be retrained. For me, they decided to *park*, by holding onto other muscles. I was not going to give in to them, so I had to figure out the best way forward, with a therapist's guidance. I must add here that everyone's physical exercises will be different, so you will need to know the appropriate exercises for you.

The following exercises were given to me by my physiotherapist, and they come in 2 stages.

Stage 1 – Massage

This stage is the beginning of visual signs that the nerve is sending messages to the affected side of the face. These exercises should be carried out when there are signs such as the nerves sending messages. Having said that, the massage must be gentle to start with.

Recovery

Using the fingers, massage and gently stretch the skin from the corner of the mouth towards the ear, and then down to the jaw bone, in a circular motion. This action can be carried out on the chin and forehead.

Gently tap the skin with the finger tips on the cheek area.

Stage 2 – Exercises

It is best to carry these out in front of a mirror, and focus on the muscles that are trying to move. These should be done in short sessions, 2–3 times daily.

Raise the eyebrows in a look of surprise, but avoid moving the corner of the mouth upwards. Then, smile, as if saying, "eee."

Wrinkle the forehead into a frown, and close the eyes slowly.

Then, wrinkle up the nose as if you smell something horrible. Following this, open your mouth wide, as if to say, "ahh." With this, pucker the lips and push forwards, as if to say, "ooo." Smile, without showing your teeth; then smile, showing teeth.

Finally, puff the cheeks out with air, and hold the lips shut so that no air escapes. It should be held for 3–5 seconds. Then, compress the lips together. After this, practise reading and speaking out loud, and at the same time, make sure to carefully sound out the words. Chewing gum must be avoided because this will exercise the wrong muscles. This takes us to the next page, to look at how your health is your wealth.

Chapter 10

Your Health Is Your Wealth

"Health is the greatest gift; contentment is the greatest wealth...."

Holistic Health

Throughout my writing, I examined areas of life, including the mind, the body, and the spirit. I also showed how they interact with the environment. With such an interaction, it is the greatest gift to our health, because our health is our wealth. Having said that, the interaction within the environment is a crucial way to monitor our well-being, on a variety of levels.

For Malcolm X, *"the future belongs to those who prepare for it today."* Indeed, we must prepare ourselves holistically, because it is natural for our body to heal itself. Being prepared for such a process can occur, even without the instructions from a doctor. The interesting thing that Malcolm X tells us is that we need to prepare for our health. But there are many variables outside the physical needs of our body, which plays a crucial role in controlling the quality of our life. Some of these controlling variables have an impact on the physical health in the environment. There is the lacking of education, stress, crime, being unemployed, divorce, lack of nutrition, and poverty. Therefore, when we are looking at the holistic health, it is significant to consider these variables and, at the same time, focus on the mind, the body, and the spirit.

Since "health is the greatest gift...," to be completely healthy, we must create and achieve that balance within. Ultimately, we are responsible for our personal health care. Once this is being taken care of, then the healing process will truly begin to take place. In addition to this, we are all different, with unique qualities, so if a health treatment works for an individual, it does not mean the same one will work for everyone. Having said that, we must be true to ourselves, because the ways we value who we are affect our health, and therefore should be a part of the healing process. Let us turn the page and look at the meaning of health.

What Is Health?

Health is a necessary component of staying in touch with your body, your emotions, and your sense of connection to things in nature. It is the state of being in control of the physical, emotional, and social aspects of health. It should not be judged entirely on the absence of an acute or a chronic illness.

Saying that, we must be mindful throughout our daily tasks, such as observing people and listening to their dialogue, to get a feel of who they are. It is also necessary to surround yourself with people who are not *toxic* in their thinking, so that your thoughts and attitudes can be healthy.

Wealth

"Nobody can give you freedom. Nobody can give you equality or justice or anything...you take it."
Malcolm X.

Even when "you take it," people's health influences their wealth. The thing that I learnt is that ill health can prevent a person from undertaking paid employment, therefore reducing their income.

Chronic ill health in childhood can affect educational outcomes. As a result, it may influence employment opportunities and earning prospects in later life. Other subtle mechanisms may play a more significant part in people's health. I have seen an increase in obesity, and autism, which is a mental condition present in very young children. I would say that parents' income influences their children's health, so children's health influences their earning when they become employable. Surely, these can influence economic outcomes, such as adults being employed, which may impact upon opportunities.

Let us now look at how healing the body through music can be essential to our lives, and is a part of our development.

Healing The Body Through Music

Just like when we breathe in and out, music has a similar effect, because it has rhythm, tension, and release. Hearing the sounds of our breath, I would say they are musical expressions. I grew up listening to a wide range of music, and because of this, I incorporate sound healing into my daily activities. Music helps me to reconnect deeply to my higher self. There is no other medium that can transport our thinking and our physical body beyond who we are. Can you think of a person who does not feel a deep connection to music?

Being in the lowest ebb of my life recently, listening to music has helped to restore my doubts and fears. It showed me a deeper understanding of the true path of my inner journey.

Whilst listening to music, it makes me feel like I am floating around in the soft, fluffy clouds. With this in mind, music can be a chemical catalyst in our brain, which releases adrenaline and endorphins, affecting both the body and the mind. It makes you feel good. This feeling is a healthy functioning of the central nervous system, because it has an effect on our emotions, our perception, and our movement. When any types of music are created from the heart, and with a purpose, it is a spiritual expression of nature.

When we listen to Bob Marley's music, such as, "Three Little Birds," and the secret language of the song, we begin to understand that this type of music is from a spiritual source, which is healing. Listening to music like this represents our response to reality.

For me, it brings clarity and coherence, and a deep personal reflection. Because there are signposts that Bob points to, they are like spiritual paths through his lyrics, and these can further shape our lives. Every day, most of us are in search of something; it might be how you are going to be creative, to the healing of a particular area in your body. Therefore, every action, and the words we say, has a sound that resonates and vibrates. This is why healing the body through positive music is so powerful.

Healthy Food

Since Bell's palsy is caused by an inflammation that decreases the blood flow to the bony canal in the skull beneath the ear, it made sense for me to increase my intake of foods rich in anti-inflammatory substances, to help deal with the swelling in the left side of my face. I included plenty of green leafy vegetables, such as spinach, kale, cabbage, asparagus, collard greens, and broccoli. I also added the vitamin family, which is known to help support nerve cell activity, and for the body to stay healthy and to grow. Vitamins are essential because they help to improve the immune and digestive processes in the body. Here are some of the members of the vitamin family.

Vitamin B6

Eat oily fish, such as salmon I aim to have it at least twice a week, because it is said to be particularly rich in omega-3 fatty acids, which we cannot make.

Vitamin B9

This vitamin may also help with nerve and muscle function by regulating the flow of energy in and out of the muscles. Eating a wide range of greens daily, and the occasional pulses, such as lentils and beans, are necessary as part of the vitamin family.

Vitamin B12

This vitamin is essential for the manufacture of red blood cells and the normal functioning of nerve cells. My food had a combination of natural yogurt, fresh sardines, avocado, and a small portion of sweet potatoes.

Some other food that I eat, are quinoa, amaranth, spelt, and rye.

Finally, to optimize your health, it is crucial to consume a well-balanced diet daily.

Food To Avoid

A lot of our food does not create a balance. I must point out here that some food we consume is healthier in quality than other types. While some people might be eating to survive, they may eat anything that they can get hold of. Why would you buy and eat any food that does not have nutritional value? As I mentioned, in depleted soils, poor-quality soil relies heavily on synthetic fertiliser products. Do we really know exactly what is in our food?

When I was a very young child, my Grandma Aunty Jenny would store tinned food in preparation for when it was needed, especially when there was a natural phenomenon, like a flood. Saying this, most food have genetically modified organisms (GMO), and Monosodium Glutamate (MSG), which means they are altered chemically through using genetic techniques. It makes no sense, that whilst my grandma was storing food for emergencies, it was also poisoning her family.

Food that contain heavy metals and pesticides can weaken the immune system, which then leads to diseases. You would have thought that during an emergency, food should have contained strong immune ingredients that Mother Earth provided, without toxic pesticides.

For me, it appears that the food industry, which includes the big names, are marketing their products with GMOs and other toxic substances and food additives. These toxic ingredients seem to be the cheapest ones available.

In my quest to find high nutrient density organic food, which I would consider suitable for my holistic health, was extremely difficult to find. Therefore, I avoid white salt, and use Himalayan salt, which has minerals found in the water of the ocean. The fact that white salt is unhealthy, I also avoid refined food, such as white bread, pastas, sugar, fried food, doughnuts, pastries, and soft drinks. Basically, I try my hardest to stay away from food that have GMOs, MSG, and other toxic ingredients, including preservatives and artificial colours. As Dr. Edward Group III reminds us, *"By cleansing your body on a regular basis, and eliminating as many toxins as possible from your environment, your body can begin to heal itself, prevent disease, and become stronger and more resilient than you ever dreamed possible!"*

About The Author

Bernice Gayle was born in Jamaica, from African parents. She grew up with her grandmother, from the age of five to twelve. Most of her spiritual journey was guided by her. At the age of twelve, Bernice Gayle joined her mother in London. Currently, she lives in London with her family. She likes to highlight the spiritual journey, such as the mind, the body, and the spirit, which we all need to be aware of.

The author is available to deliver presentations to appropriate audiences. You can contact the author directly for rates and availability, at successwithbellspalsy.com.

To order more books, please visit:
Pempamsie Bookshop, 102 Brixton Hill, London SW2 1AH
Maa Maat Centre, 366A High Rd, Tottenham, N17 9HT

Finally, if this book has awakened your spiritual journey, then you can invite others to feel the energy and the vibration that you encountered. Feeling these, you should pass the book on.

www.ingramcontent.com/pod-product-compliance
Lightning Source LLC
Chambersburg PA
CBHW071404220526
45469CB00004B/1156